Stammering

DAVID COMPTON

A stammerer since early childhood, David Compton was born in London in 1930. At the age of ten he composed a short verse about a snowdrop, now mercifully lost, shortly after which he declared his intention of becoming a writer. Since then he has published a couple of dozen novels, has written plays for radio and television, and has worked as an editor for many publishers, including the *Reader's Digest*. He is married, with children and grand-children. Following a number of itinerant years, he now lives again in London, very close to the streets of his youth.

A.D. 1913. May 1. No. 10,256.
SAMUEL'S Complete Specification.

(1 SHEET)

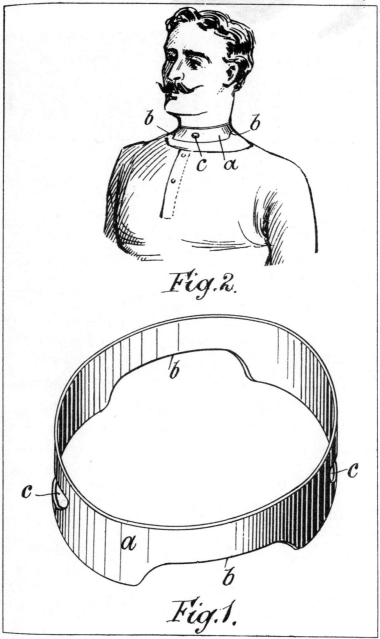

Fig.2.

Fig.1.

Stammering

ITS NATURE, HISTORY, CAUSES AND CURES

David Compton

Hodder & Stoughton
LONDON SYDNEY AUCKLAND

British Library Cataloguing in Publication Data

Compton, David
Stammering
I. Title
616.85

ISBN 0-340-56274-9 ✓

First published in Great Britain 1993

Illustrations facing pages 20 and 21 are reproduced
by kind permission of the Bodleian Library: John Johnson Collection

Published by Hodder and Stoughton,
a division of Hodder and Stoughton Ltd,
Mill Road, Dunton Green,
Sevenoaks, Kent TN13 2YA
Editorial Office: 47 Bedford Square,
London WC1B 3DP

Photoset by Rowland Phototypesetting Ltd,
Bury St Edmunds, Suffolk

Printed in Great Britain by
Clays Ltd, St Ives plc

Contents

1
Why this book?

. . . the people around me didn't know my ugly secret . . .

In recent years stammering has received good media coverage. It's no longer one of those disabilities nobody talks about. Stammerers have appeared on television discussing their difficulties; sympathetic, well-informed articles have appeared in the press; fluent public figures have revealed their secret battles with disfluency. The subject, one might think, has been pretty well run into the ground.

So why this book?

Because it's needed. Because most media coverage of complex subjects, no matter how well-intentioned, ends up raising many more questions than it answers. Because misapprehensions easily creep in. Because media coverage isn't available for reference all in one place.

Stammers are confusing afflictions. For one thing, no two stammers are the same. For another, no one stammer is the same all the time. Stammering therapies come in a confusing number of shapes and sizes and suggested causes range from brindled cats at cock-crow to anal-retentive avoidance behaviours. There's even confusion, at least in the English language, as to when a stammer's a stammer and when it's really a stutter.

When I was growing up I (and many of the people I have talked to) believed that a stammer was the humming sort of stuff I did on 'm's and 'n's, and a stutter was the exploding sort of stuff I did on 't's and 'b's. Not so. In fact, according to the dictionary, the difference between hums and explosions isn't one that the non-stammering, non-stuttering world has got round to. Historically, stammer and stutter mean the same thing, and have been in use for centuries. Stutter appeared in the fifteenth century as a shorter word, to 'stut', but stammerers seem always to have suffered polysyllabically. The two words were more or less interchangeable until the mid-nineteenth century, when they became separated on a national and cultural basis – stutter being used more in the United States and stammer in Britain.

Nowadays, instead of either expression you may hear of *dysphemia*. This sounds horribly like in-group medical jargon, another of those new, fancy words invented by experts in order to smarten up old, unfancy afflictions. In fact – as I'll explain in Chapter 4 – I don't think it's so bad: dysphemia has come into use in connection with some excellent recent American research and it's the product of refreshing new thinking.

There's also CPSDS, a long string of initials for people who like long strings of initials. It stands for *Chronic Perseverative Speech Disfluency Syndrome*. This, too, I'll be getting to later. Surprisingly, it also turns out to have a lot more to be said in its favour than you might think.

They all mean much the same thing, of course: making a bloody fool of yourself every time you open your bloody mouth. That's what this book is about – about how and why and when and who, about stammer therapies, and about the ways (often unhelpful) in which nice ordinary people deal with the stammerers they meet.

Nice ordinary people ... it's a phrase I'll use a lot in this book. It signifies for me an entire longed-for, unattainable world. When I was a child, a teenager, a young man, there were many things I wanted: a shunting engine for my train set, a Norton motor bike, a successful career as a writer. But more than any of these I wanted to be a nice ordinary person. Maybe I never formulated it in so many words, but as an idea it was always with me. Walking down the street, sitting on a bus, lying on the beach, standing in a lift, I remember being pleased that the people around me didn't know my ugly secret. To them I looked just like anybody else. They were nice ordinary people. If they thought about me at all, they thought I was like them. I wasn't. I was a stammerer.

Now, many years later, I've mostly come to terms with stammering. And indeed the stammer itself has mercifully become more manageable. But it still trips me up when I most don't want it to. And there's still the difference, that uncomfortable, dangerous, unpredictable difference, between me before I've spoken – a nice ordinary person – and me after I've spoken – a stammerer.

Don't worry. This isn't going to be an autobiography, the story of my stammering life. Such books are already available, many of them well worth reading, and I doubt if there's much I could add to them. Certainly I've done nothing that I believe other stammerers could learn from. No – as promised, this book will simply try to get all the facts together, and to explain the stammerer and his world; not as a plea for more public sympathy, nor even for more public money (although where treatment for children is concerned that would always be welcome), but in the cause of better understanding. Stammerers' better understanding of themselves, and non-stammerers' better understanding of ways in which they can, at the very least, avoid worsening the stammerer's burden.

But first, an old joke. A man visits his GP about his severe stammer. The doctor sits him down and says to him, 'Tell me about your speech problem.' He glances at his watch. 'And make it snappy.'

An old joke? Old maybe, but still alive and kicking. Snappiness is as desirable as it ever was. In fact, more so. A friend of mine was very recently reminded of that, when she was in her local supermarket . . .

She likes supermarkets. She functions very well in them. She even buys her bread in them. Granary. It's not as good as the bread from the baker at the end of her street, but there she has to buy wholemeal. She'd much rather have granary, and the baker at the end of her street makes a beauty of a loaf, but with him she has to ask for it, and the 'g' is too much for her blocks and twitches, so she sticks with safe old ho-ho-wholemeal. In supermarkets she can buy all the granary she wants, no hassle.

So she was in her supermarket. She'd filled her basket and she was waiting at the check-out. While she waited she passed her time reading the guff on the covers of the women's magazines on the rack – no-fail cake recipes, pain-less diets, how to satisfy your man. Suddenly she spotted a new one: *Fifty Ways of Doing Almost Anything Faster.*

Hurry, hurry, hurry . . . She had to laugh.

I had to laugh too, when she told me, but it wasn't funny. Is that what today's magazine readers really want? The magazine's editor thought so. Personally, I'd buy a magazine that promised me *Fifty Excuses for Doing Just About Everything More Slowly*. That way I might actually get around to saying what needed saying.

I don't suggest that stammerers are alone in feeling put-upon these days. Anybody with less than the expected rapidity in thought, word or deed has a hard time. Stammerers are just one group among many.

And besides, as I've already admitted, stammerers get plenty of sympathy. This is the age of special interest groups. Maybe the public's had enough of them. Wasn't there an interview with a stammerer in that colour supplement only last month? And wasn't one of them doing his embarrassing thing on that morning chat show, whatever it's called? For heaven's sake, haven't you heard of compassion fatigue?

I don't want to sound ungrateful – I'm *not* ungrateful – and I *have* heard of compassion fatigue. And yes, stammerers *do* get public sympathy, thanks mostly to the Association For Stammerers, which does a fine job of getting stammering talked about sympathetically in this country. Similar organisations do good work across continental Europe, and there's another in the United States, called the Stutter Project. But sympathy is only a beginning, and it's often a substitute for action.

Parents with stammering children need more than sympathy, they need help. So do severe adult stammerers, and the nice ordinary people who sometimes have to listen to stammerers. But before help can be successful, there has to be understanding.

Everybody knows at least one stammerer. In Britain alone there are over half a million. Stammerers make up at least one in a hundred of the world's population. Among young children that figure rises to five in a hundred. These are worldwide statistics. There isn't a culture, there isn't a language group, there isn't a nation on the face of the earth that doesn't have its stammerers. One Japanese man was so shamed by his condition that he burnt down the ancient Temple of the Golden Pavilion as a public sign of his despair.

An Arab told his therapist, 'Women take their children and flee in mortal terror when they hear me stammer.' In West Africa, Bantu men traditionally treat their stammers by chewing garlic . . .

There have been decades of research into the affliction, much of it very technical, some of it contradictory, all of it inconclusive. For example, four out of five stammerers are male – many explanations are offered for this but none can be generally agreed upon.

Stammering remains one of the least understood of human disorders – by the experts, by the general public, and by stammerers themselves. In this book I hope to cut away some of the clutter, to summarise current thinking and the reasoning behind it, and to set stammering in the widest possible context, social and historical as well as medical and scientific. There are things to be learnt about any disorder, simply by examining changing attitudes towards it.

Incidentally, from now on I shall refer to the genus *stammerer* as 'he'. This isn't sexism, it's for simplicity's sake, in recognition of the high percentage of stammerers who are men. By the same reasoning I shall refer to the genus *therapist* as 'she': there are many more female therapists than male. The English language doesn't cope well with he/she, him/her, hers/his.

This book is not a self-help manual. Several of these are available and they'll be discussed in due course. Neither will it be a list of stammerers' horror stories – who needs it? But I also don't intend to try to whitewash the disorder: little is gained by understatement and much may be lost.

As a group, stammerers try to emphasise the positive. This is understandable. They like to cheer each other up. Here in Britain the quarterly magazine of the Association For Stammerers, *Speaking Out*, provides a forum for brisk, affirmative stammerers who look determinedly on the bright side, encouraging their less extrovert fellows. This is fine within the stammering community, but it gives outsiders a false picture. The PR stammerers too, the front men interviewed on radio or television, are always well adjusted and coherent. The less well adjusted and the less coherent members of the great majority tend to stay at home, keeping their heads down and their mouths shut.

In the first few months of my research for this book I visited several stammerers' support groups at which the members, sure of a patient hearing, spoke out boldly. They were an impressive lot. I travelled round the country also, interviewing stammerers, all of whom seemed to be leading successful, well-rounded lives. And I read up on famous stammerers of the past – they too had refused to let their handicap get in their way.

There's been a surprisingly large number of well-known stammering authors. Starting my collection with Virgil, I allowed in Erasmus, then moved on a few centuries to Charles Darwin, Charles Lamb, Lewis Carroll, Charles Kingsley, Leigh Hunt, Ronald Firbank, Arnold Bennett, Somerset Maugham, Aldous Huxley, Kenneth Tynan, Elizabeth Bowen, Patrick Campbell, Margaret Drabble, Philip Larkin, Monica Furlong, Ray Connolly . . . So many of them – could there be a genetic predisposition among writers to stammer? Or was it just that stammerers turned to writing out of sheer desperation?

Apparently not. Arriving at the present, I discovered that plenty of them turned to acting instead. Very casual research produced Marilyn Monroe, Frankie Howerd, Jonathan Miller, Rowan Atkinson, Derek Nimmo. And then there was Winston Churchill, a writer, and theatrical too . . .

In short, the world was full of confident, successful stammerers. So why all the fuss? At worst, stammering seemed to be little more than an inconvenience – and even then, an inconvenience less to the stammerer than to his listener. Which of course, for the majority of stammerers, is wicked nonsense.

The truth is, stammering is hell, and the worse the stammer the worse the hell. The stammerer intends to say something, but instead his mouth jerks, his face screws up, and he makes demented noises. It doesn't always happen, but he can be sure it will happen whenever he least wants it to. He tries to stop it and he fails. He fails grossly and he fails publicly. He has a picture of himself and it's ugly.

The personal outrage that chronic stammerers endure cannot be overstated. They are shaped and completely dominated by their disability. One American sufferer, Wendell

Johnson, who became an influential speech therapist in the 1930s, wrote this: 'I am a stutterer. I am not like other people. I must think differently, act differently, live differently. Like other stutterers, other exiles, I have known all my life a great sorrow and a great hope together, and they have made me the kind of person I am.'

The assault is threefold, upon the stammerer's integrity as a sentient, self-willed and self-aware individual, upon his self-image, and upon the image he presents to the outside world. If he persistently cannot prevent himself from doing something he knows to be painful and destructive, that puts his integrity into serious question. If he persistently behaves in an ugly, alienating fashion, he acquires the self-image of someone who is ugly and alienated. And if he persistently fails to communicate verbally in a society in which verbal communication is just about all anybody has, then the identity he presents is that of a tense, unattractive person, troublesome and probably stupid.

The speech-impaired child experiences these assaults also. His words, which are his richest, most exciting contact point with life and love and learning, become a struggle, a source of constant anxiety. His disfluencies may well conceal his intelligence and hamper his progress at school. They will certainly expose him to ridicule. Inevitably, although bruised and full of dread, most children will learn to get by. They're great survivors. But someone far wiser than I has already pointed out that the child is father to the man. The bruised child, full of dread, is the bruised man, and his dread has grown with the years, reinforced by bitter experience.

These are unattractive facts. If the stammerer admits them it's bad for morale and sounds like self-pity. And if the non-stammerer admits them he or she might feel bound to do something. And for *do something*, friends, read spend public money.

Obviously, all guardians of public purses have to establish priorities. The stammerer recognises that his affliction, which isn't infectious, or life-threatening, or even all that unsightly, must expect a place well down the list. Exactly how far down, though, has never been properly argued. Dr Eugene Cooper, who is a distinguished speech therapist from

Alabama in the United States, reports that his state appor-
tions its health care funds according to a list of fourteen
classifications. And guess where stammering comes on that
list. No – not at the bottom. Not quite. In fact, stammering
comes one up from the bottom, outdone in unimportance
only by 'other minor disorders'.

It's not necessarily that Alabamans have it in for stammerers. They may well just be responding to the affirmative
self-image stammerers present. In the course of arguing
one's case, maybe one can be *too* affirmative.

In Britain the National Health Service has never listed its
priorities so openly. But British speech therapists will tell
you not only that there's unreasonable variation from region
to region in the support they get, but also that the general
level of funding is lamentable. They would, of course. No
worker in a country's social services has ever been known
to say that his or her level of funding *isn't* lamentable. Even
so, international medical opinion seems to agree that there
should be on average twenty-six qualified speech therapists
per one hundred thousand people, and in Britain there are
fewer than six. And there is undeniable evidence of this
disparity in the long waiting-lists that face speech-impaired
children urgently in need of help, which is particularly dis-
turbing since these are the stammerers most likely to respond
to treatment if caught young enough.

Everybody knows there'll never be enough money for
everything. But when the disparity between funding and
need is as desperate as that which British therapists face
(their salary scales are scandalously low too), then this may
partly be a result of the fine job stammerers do of playing
down their disability. So it's high time someone played them
up. If there aren't any votes in stammering, there bloody
well ought to be.

This, then, is a book written on behalf of the enforcedly
silent majority. Few stammerers are as confident and clever
and sexy as Dr Jonathan Miller. This is a book written on
behalf of the shy, the embarrassed, the frustrated, the afraid,
the undervalued, the discriminated-against, all the men and
women whose careers are blighted by their disability, whose
relationships are circumscribed, whose lives centre round

the need to survive from one stammering situation to the next, men and women who would never dare to speak on radio or television, and who would certainly never dream of letting themselves be interviewed by some damfool writer like me.

And finally in this chapter, for the benefit of fluent speakers, I want to try to capture on the page what stammering actually feels like. Different stammerers inevitably come up with different descriptions – the transfer from feelings to words is always difficult, especially from feelings so intense and traumatic, and so mysterious – but when fluent speakers see a stammerer struggling I think it would be helpful if they had some sort of picture of what's going on, or at least of what he thinks is going on. Such a description may also throw useful light on the success of some therapies and the failure of others. I'm not sure that researchers have always asked the right questions of stammerers before they've proposed their cures and causes.

A metaphor is needed, and the metaphor that seems best to match the subjective experience of stammerers I've talked to involves a snake – a snake of the crushing sort, a python or a boa constrictor, that is felt to be living in what I'll call the house of their speech.

Everybody, fluent or disfluent, has this house: it's the part of their minds where their speech is stored, the house they have to visit when they need to collect words and sentences for talking. The house has many rooms: rooms where different subjects are kept, rooms that are familiar and rooms that are half-forgotten, rooms that communicate particular atmospheres and rooms that answer to particular moods . . . And when fluent people are talking they move calmly through the rooms in their house, picking out the words they need, using them, putting them back ready for the next time. Once in a while the shelves are in a mess and the right word gets mislaid, or maybe the atmosphere in the room is uneasy, and then people hesitate, repeat themselves, even go back and start again. But usually their stock of words is in its right place and their journey through the house is smooth and steady.

Stammerers, on the other hand, seem to have a snake living in the house of their speech, a serpent that follows them from room to room. It's a malignant creature, quite merciless, watching for the smallest opportunity to humiliate them. It trips them when it can, threatens them, lies silkily along the shelves, darts out to crush their hearts and paralyse their lungs, or forces itself up their throats to strangle them. Sometimes – if they tiptoe, if they go very carefully, if it's their lucky day – sometimes the serpent is dozing, or waiting for them in another room, and they get by without alerting it. Sometimes the serpent is expecting them to take a certain word and they fool it by taking another. Sometimes they manage to beat it down by the sheer strength of their will-power. Sometimes they disguise themselves and get on nicely for a while because the serpent doesn't recognise them. But it's always around somewhere, lurking, ready to dash out, and it's pretty damn clever.

I'm sure this sounds fanciful, melodramatic, but I promise you it's fair. Above all, it captures the essentially inner and alien nature of a stammer. The outward frustrations it brings are finally nothing beside the inner fury and self-disgust, the despair, the sheer *exhaustion* that comes from resisting alien muscles that grip you, an alien malevolence that mocks you, an alien force that possesses you.

In actual fact, of course, that's all nonsense. There's nothing alien, only the stammerer. There's no alien force out there, no alien force in here. The stammer is the stammerer. The stammerer is his stammer. But that's not an observation that seems to help much. Does he want to be told he is his stammer? Does he want to be reminded, every time he stammers, that there's nothing and nobody else involved, he's doing it to himself? Does he hell.

So much for facts and understanding. They're seldom comfortable, but they're all we have.

Interestingly, since I wrote the above, serendipity has struck. For a more poetic, more powerful understanding of what stammering is, a stammering friend down in Devon has drawn my attention to a passage in Nietzsche's remarkable book, *Thus Spake Zarathustra*. In it the philosopher sage who's telling the story has a hideous vision. This is how the episode is presented in A. Tille's translation from the original German:

And, verily, the sight I saw, its like I had never seen. I saw a young Shepherd, writhing, choking, quivering, with face distorted, from whose mouth a black and heavy snake hung down.

Saw I ever so much loathing and wan horror in one face? My hand tore at the serpent and tore – in vain! I could not tear the serpent from his throat. Then a voice within me cried: Bite! Bite!

Bite off its head! Bite! – thus cried the voice of my horror, my hate, my loathing, my pity, all the good and evil in me cried out . . .

The Shepherd bit, as my cry counselled him: he bit with all his strength! He spat the snake's head far from him – then up he sprang, no longer a shepherd, no longer a man, but one transfigured, light-encompassed, one that laughed! . . .

In the book Zarathustra implores the gods for an explanation of his vision. I can give him one. If any stammerer could bite off the head of his stammer and spit it from him, he too would be one transfigured, light-encompassed, one who laughed . . .

~

From *The Stammerer's Complaint*, 1834

Oh! tis a sore affliction, to restrain
From mere necessity, the glowing thought;
To feel the fluent cataract of speech
Check'd by some wintry spell, and frozen up,
Just as it leapeth from the precipice!
To be the butt of wordy captious fools,
And see the sneering self-complacent smile
Of victory on their lips, when I might prove,
(But for some little word I dare not utter)
That innate truth is not a specious lie;
To hear foul slander blast an honour'd name,
Yet breathe no fact to drive the fiend away;
To mark neglected virtue in the dust,
Yet have no word to pity or console;
To feel just indignation swell my breast,
Yet know the fountain of my wrath is seal'd;
To see my fellow-mortals hurrying on
Down the steep cliff of crime, down to perdition,
Yet have no voice to warn, no voice to win!

'Tis to be mortified in every point,
Baffled at every turn of life, for want
Of that most common privilege of man,
The merest drug of gorged society,
Words, – windy words.

Martin Tupper

2
History

. . . the therapeutic value of pebbles is not to be mocked . . .

Any useful account of the history of stammering has to begin at the beginning, with the history of speech, because it's early on in that, just past the grunt and grab stage, that the seeds of disfluency were sown.

It's humankind's ability to speak, more than any other ability, that separates us from the rest of the animal kingdom. Obviously, in evolutionary terms our way with words gave us enormous advantages. First of all, the archaeological record suggests an efficient uniformity of tool design that would have been virtually impossible to achieve without language, simply by example. Then again, we clearly needed language for essential co-operative enterprises such as fire-keeping and the hunting of large animals. Although all primates, including *Homo sapiens*, use visual communication – facial expressions, gestures, shrugs – as well as non-linguistic screams and cries, only we have been able to employ sounds as open symbols, able to be recombined to relay an infinite variety of messages.

Even so, many scientists believe that the power of speech – or more precisely, the power of language (and not for nothing is the word 'power' used here) – has done something far more fundamental than simply enable us to conceive of poems and space stations. They suggest that the development of language went hand in hand with, and was in fact essential to, the evolution of the human brain itself, and therefore of the human mind.

With its ability to handle abstractions, speech frees us from the tyranny of the moment. It lets us organise experience,

13

relate past to present to future, wander at will. Memory of one kind or another is possessed by all sensate life forms, but for as long as it's stored away non-linguistically, in the form of images or sensations, it seems to be available only when stimulated and brought into consciousness by similar images or sensations. All the evidence suggests that a cat sitting in the sun thinks only of sitting in the sun. A discrete event is needed, a hunger pang or a rustling leaf, before other mental activities can be stimulated, and for performing such straightforward, one-at-a-time tasks the cat's small brain is admirably sufficient.

On the other hand, if memories are to be retrieved on demand, and manipulated, related to one another in the manner that produces not just responses to the moment but consecutive rational thought, then a far more complex mechanism is needed — one that can store material in the form of abstract symbols. In short, words are needed. Words, strung together into language, are the cataloguers of our brain's resources, our guide through them, and our wonderfully versatile retrieval system.

Modern man, *Homo sapiens*, has a brain almost twice the size of his immediate predecessor, *Homo erectus*, whose smaller brain volume apparently remained constant (and therefore presumably adequate to his needs) for around a million years. Most of modern man's extra brain capacity, acquired since then, seems to be involved in sentence-forming and speech-understanding activities. It's as if, once the language breakthrough indicated by the archaeological record had occurred, its demands were insatiable. It would actively have sought new connections, actively created new channels, as language does today, and would plausibly have instigated precisely the developments in brain capacity down the millennia that palaeontologists have found. It seems, in fact, that the two large grey squashy hemispheres of the cerebral cortex that today lie over the small, far older reptilian cerebellum could not have developed to their present size and complexity without language to spur them on, to force the changes, to demand ever greater resources of storage and interaction.

It's difficult to say how long this process took. The only clues lie in the fossil record. To achieve reasonable voice production we now know that a high roof to the mouth is necessary, and this doesn't begin to appear in fossil remains until around a million and a half years ago. Laryngeal developments can be detected at about this time also, but both these changes are very slight, and open to argument, and they really don't prove much. Modern speech may well be no more than 100,000 years old, for only by then does our knowledge of brain structure tell us that the left hemisphere had become specialised for language, and that there were areas of brain cells, fanning back from behind the left ear, that linked it with the visual cortex at the back of the head. Thus the basic ability to attach verbal meaning to visual images was made possible, and with it sophistications such as reading – first the reading of signs, animal spoor, cloud formations, arrow marks drawn in the sand, and eventually of written words.

(Pictorial art, interestingly, is an even more recent acquisition, if the short, 20,000 year-old record of cave paintings is anything to go by.)

The relevance of all this to stammering lies in the recent nature of speech as a human ability, located in the cerebral cortex but possessing close interconnections with the much older, less 'reasonable' cerebellum, centre of the limbic system which, although primitive, is still the brain's chief arousal mechanism. Speech demonstrably taxes the capacities of our brains to the utmost – and sometimes beyond what they can deal with. Its mechanisms are new in evolutionary terms, delicate, and uniquely complex. Thus it is in a patient's uncertainties of speech volume, pitch or intensity that Parkinson's disease and other lower motor neurone disturbances first show themselves. It is in uncertainties of breathing, articulation and word retrieval that the limbic system most often interferes when it expresses its owner's fear, rage, love, hate. And it is in the total loss of the power of speech that many physical or emotional traumas find their first and most significant outlet.

So were there Stone Age stammerers? I can only answer that there's no evidence that there weren't, and quite good reasons to suppose that there were. Certainly the condition isn't restricted today to what we arrogantly call our 'advanced' societies – less 'advanced' countries have their fair share of stammerers. Experts tell us that around 1½ per cent of the world's population currently stammers, and that's a cross-cultural figure. Local conditions may temporarily enlarge it – the high-stress societies of Japan and the United States are showing higher percentages just at present – but a 1½ per cent overall rate seems plausible, and can be corroborated at least for the hundred years or so of our clinical records. And before that there's ample evidence that stammerers were around to a significant degree.

As far back as 2,500 years ago the Chinese poet Laotze mentioned stammering in one of his poems. The next documented example seems to occur around 1200 BC, and appears in the second book of the Judaeo-Christian bible, when the Jewish God is calling upon Moses to lead his chosen people, the Israelites, out of the wilderness. Poor Moses had his doubts: 'O my Lord,' he says in the King James version, 'I am not eloquent . . . I am slow of speech and of a slow tongue . . .' His Lord's sensible response to this is to appoint Moses' older brother Aaron as his spokesperson.

Admittedly this isn't much of a basis for claiming that Moses was a stammerer, and biblical scholars have suggested that the text in fact refers to his difficulty, as a man educated by the Egyptian ruling class, with the Hebrew language (tongue) of the people he was being asked to lead. But further digging produces a passage in the Koran where Moses – a respected Islamic prophet – features at his prayers: 'O Lord, unloose thou the knot in my tongue, that the people may understand my saying . . .' This doesn't sound like a linguistic difficulty. The key word here is 'knot' – a knotted tongue has long been a popular image for the stammer. Nothing whatever to do with Moses' problems with Hebrew irregular verbs.

In the light of this, Moses' first remark, 'I am not eloquent', sounds like an oddly familiar understatement, as charming and tactful as the comment often made by worried parents today, 'My boy's not good at talking.'

Furthermore, a few pages later Moses is addressing his people fluently and directly, without his brother as intermediary, and this seems much more likely to be a stammering remission brought about by his new and improved self-image as his God's appointed, than the result of private lessons in colloquial Hebrew.

By the time of the ancient Greeks, stammering was clearly a commonplace. Herodotus wrote of it in 400 BC, and Aristotle a hundred years later. And the most famous stammerer of all time has to be poor young Demosthenes, who was successfully treated for his condition by the actor Satyrus . . . although even here there are sour-pusses who try to tell us it was only his voice production that was poor, or his intonation. But the therapy described – orating with his mouth filled with pebbles and running up steep hills carrying heavy weights – sounds a bit drastic for such a minor problem.

Incidentally, Satyrus must have been one of the first in a long, slightly disreputable line of theatrical folk turned therapists that has continued well into this century. He seems to have known his job, though – Demosthenes went on to become a very successful public speaker. The therapeutic value of pebbles is not to be mocked, nor that of hard labour on hillsides. Indeed, as this book will show, there are very few therapies, very few behaviour modifications, no matter how bizarre, that haven't helped stammerers at one time or another.

Another Greek stammerer, name of Bataros, resorted in his anguish to the oracle at Delphi for advice. She recommended exile to a far foreign land, which suggests that there may have been political overtones to the case that have got lost in the transmission. Certainly he pushed off to North Africa where the change of air – or something – was so helpful that he was able to become governor of Cirene. He also gave his name, if unwittingly, to his own particular brand of stammer – first syllable repetitions – for they were known in medieval times as 'batarismus'.

The Romans were so familiar with, and so unembarrassed by, stammering (poor Claudius's, for one) that there's even a Roman family name, Balbus, that refers to the affliction. Similarly the ninth century saw a Frankish king who was popularly known as Ludwig the Stammerer.

By that time, of course, stammering was well established in the medical lexicon, both in Europe and across the Bosphorus, where Avicenna, the Arabian doctor and poet (a pleasantly frequent combination in those days) wrote in some detail of the condition, its causes and treatments. But this was tame stuff. It was the renowned Greek physician Galen who recommended that the tongues of stammerers be soundly cauterised – thus establishing the theory of pain as the great redeemer that persisted for many centuries, probably finding its apogee among the exultantly punitive Victorians.

Dr Mercuralis, in the 1580s, was a notable exception. He prescribed nothing more radical than a calm life, regular bowels, and vigorous exercise. Francis Bacon, too, in tune with the hedonism of his time, was an easy-going fellow. 'Divers, we see, do stut,' he wrote in the 1620s. 'The Cause may be . . . (in most) the Refrigeration of the Tongue . . . And we see, that in those that Stut, if they drink Wine moderately, they Stut lesse, because it heateth . . .' An excellent theory. The difficulty must always have been to determine whether they did indeed 'stut lesse', or were simply too drunk to care how much they bloody stutted.

As I've already said, in the history of stammering the tongue has traditionally come in for a lot of attention. A few years before Francis Bacon, a Frenchman, Guy de Chauliac, was recommending 'application of embrocation, cauteries, blisters, and gargles for the tongue'. Censoriousness was never far away. In 1700 the Swiss doctor, Konrad Amman, wrote grumpily of stammering as 'a blundering of utterance which arises from bad habit'. This was the first great age of surgery when, despite a lack of anaesthetics, antiseptics or antibiotics, cutting was perceived as a remedy for virtually anything, including bad habits: thus stammerers' frenums were severed, and tongues were either pierced with hot needles or had wedges cut from their roots. Apparently such procedures were discontinued only after word began to get about in the general public of the many patients who were dying in agony from the resulting infections and abscesses.

Over in the New World a Boston clergyman, Cotton Mather (son of the wonderfully named Increase Mather) was more merciful. Although he was a brisk man, who countenanced witchcraft trials and executions, his inoffensive 1724 remedy for stammering was: 'Use yourself to a Deliberate Way of Speaking, a Drawling that shall be little short of

Singing . . .' Clearly he'd noticed, as many others had, that no stammerer stammers when he sings.

Back in Britain, with the beginning of the nineteenth century, stammering became a growth industry. Stammering 'schools' sprang up throughout the country, public lectures linked the complaint with blushing and promised instant cures, and hardly a year passed without a new self-help book on the subject. There seem to be two possible explanations for all this activity. Either there was a sudden genuine increase in the number of stammerers needing treatment, or more probably social attitudes to speech and language hardened with the appearance of the first pronouncing dictionaries and a stable population of stammerers just got noticed more. But in either case, the principal result was the creation of a new profession – centred not only around stammering but also around the unembarrassed recognition that a man's success in life often depended on his vowels and aspirates, the class-based manner in which he spoke.

The first Englishman to describe himself as an 'elocutionist', back in the early 1800s, was almost certainly the Londoner James Thelwell. Self-trained, he was so well received by stammerers that he was able to charge seventy guineas – then a huge amount of money – for a three-month course of treatment. His writings, although secretive about the exact nature of his treatment (he had his livelihood to protect), suggest that although he was of course a disciplinarian, he was also an acute clinician who based his procedures on his own closely observed experience. Others, needless to say, were less scrupulous: in their schools the appalling stringency of the regimens seems to have been imposed upon the wretched inmates more or less for its own sake, because the spirit of the time expected it, and also, I suspect, because the 'elocutionists' enjoyed it. The cane, one gathers, was never far from their hands.

Thelwell soon became a leading figure in the battle for patients that inevitably flared up between doctors and lay elocutionists like himself. The argument centred round the exact nature of stammering, as either a medically identifiable disease (the business of doctors), or as simply a nervous – for which read *bad* – habit (fodder for elocutionists), and for a while Thelwell's side was victorious. So much so that a certain Dr William Abbotts was prompted to fulminate in the press that treatment for stammering had got into the hands of 'elocutionists ... decayed actors, mere music masters'.

This controversy persisted well into the nineteenth century – the disciplinarians, in particular, must have been reluctant to give up to the doctors what was otherwise clearly an excellent outlet for well-paid brutality. Interestingly, it was the same Dr Abbotts who published the first popular book that presented 'nerves' as the main cause of stammering, and that described sympathetically the social suffering, and even genuine ill health that was associated with the condition. His book quickly went into nine editions, which suggests that, at least among stammerers and their relatives, his message was welcomed.

Fifty years earlier, a Dr Marshall Hall, elected to the Royal Society for his work on the spinal cord, had also studied stammering as a nervous disorder and had published on the subject, but his book had probably been overshadowed at the time by his more controversial campaigning for the abolition of flogging in the British Army, and for improved public safety in railway compartments. Marshall Hall was a man of wide interests.

In passing, that was the time, 1833, when stammering made what must be its sole lasting contribution to the English language. A certain Richard Turner, Methodist, a plasterer by profession and a severe stammerer, produced the word 'teetotal' under stress during a courageous speech at a meeting of his local Temperance Society. The local press picked it up, and it stuck. I don't know if we stammerers should feel proud of the connection, but there it is.

Meanwhile, cures proliferated. Many were mechanical, gadgets to be held within the stammerer's mouth or strapped to his person. Little whistles beneath the tongue were claimed to be invaluable, as were small, very sharp gold or ivory forks (punishment again). Leather straps pressed on the Adam's apple, and others were applied to constrict the stammerer's 'excessive breathing'. A Frenchman invented what he called a 'Muthonome', to help maintain rhythmic speech: it did well but was later marketed even more successfully to musicians, under the trade name 'Metronome'.

ELOCUTION.

AT THE FREEMASONS' HALL,

BOLD-STREET, LIVERPOOL,

On Monday, 24th, Wednesday, 26th, and
Saturday, 29th January, 1803,

MR. THELWALL

WILL DELIVER THE SECOND SERIES OF HIS

COURSE OF LECTURES:

ON THE

SCIENCE AND PRACTICE

OF

ELOCUTION:

With Illustrations, Readings, and Recitals, and Strictures,
Literary and Critical, on the respective Authors,
and various styles of composition.

To begin at Seven o'Clock, and conclude at half past Nine.

---

*Transferable Tickets for the three nights, 7s.—Single ad-
mission 3s. 6d.—Social Tickets (admitting
four persons) 10s. 6d.*

Social Tickets cannot be procured at the doors; but may be had of
the Lecturer, at Mr. Brown's, No. 5, Paradise-street; and of Mr. Jones,
Mr. Robinson, Mr. Woodward, and Mr. Rushton, Booksellers; where,
also, may be had (price 6d.) *Selections* for the respective evenings.

Also, price 7s.

POEMS IN RETIREMENT,

WITH MEMOIRS OF THE LIFE OF THE AUTHOR.

J. M'Creery, Printer, Houghton-Street.

*It was in the early 19th Century that a good speaking voice first
became widely recognised as a social and professional asset*

COUNTY HALL, AYLESBURY.

MR. E. SLATTERIE

WILL DELIVER A SERIES OF

Four Lectures

ON

ELOCUTION,

AT THE COUNTY-HALL, AYLESBURY,

ON THE EVENINGS OF

Thursday 8th, Friday 9th, Tuesday 13th, and Wednesday 14th of September, 1836.

TO BEGIN PUNCTUALLY AT SEVEN.

Mr. SLATTERIE deems it requisite to state, that his object is to make himself known, throughout the country, as a Teacher of Elocution, and a Corrector of Impediments, resident in London:—he therefore seeks introduction, rather than emolument. His Lectures are not mere Recitations, but attempts to elucidate the principles and to enforce the practice of the science. At the same time, to secure interest, Mr. S. aims to convey much of the instruction, through the medium of amusement, by the graphic exhibition of Elocutionary Defects, their cause and cure; thus blending the useful with the more pleasing part of the science.

TERMS OF ADMISSION.

Single Tickets. .... 2s.
Four Tickets .... 6s.

Mr. S. will feel obliged if those who attend his Lectures will procure Tickets of Mr. May, Bookseller, or at the George Inn, Aylesbury.

INSTRUCTION in READING, ELOCUTION, and COMPOSITION.

Books of the Illustrations, Sixpence each.

Advice in Cases of Impediment.

(Town Address, 15, Paternoster Row.)

MAY, PRINTER, AYLESBURY.

By the 1830s elocutionists were already including 'Advice in Cases of Impediment' in the programme

The doctors fought back. Dr Langenbeck, in 1833, was loudly in favour of cathartic laxative, leeches on the lips, and – this is on record – eating goat faeces. While the blunt Dr Frank, thirty years later, strongly recommended 'a good flogging'.

Not only the British were punitive. The Finns concocted a vile-smelling ointment, Hirven Sarven Tippola (Elk Oil Drops), for the stammerer's throat. It was reported to be of more use rubbed on cattle to keep the flies away in summer. Nevertheless it was still available commercially as recently as 1971. Available for stammerers, that is. Not cows.

Other cures included J. H. A. Poett's 'Stammering Trumpet' (for which no description or picture survives, so that one can only guess at its operation), the application of electric shocks to the spine, and – rather charmingly – 'steaming the throat with aromatic herbs and learning the German language'.

Upper-class parents became so concerned for their sons' speech that Eton employed a residential full-time elocutionist. And for humbler folk there were the books, the lectures, and a wide range of often cut-price stammering schools. Mr Poett (of trumpet fame) ran one in London, as did Mr Alexander Ball up in Edinburgh. Benjamin Beasley, in Birmingham, was very successful with the 'Beasley System', invented by his father, a stammerer and wealthy armaments manufacturer.[1] Beasley Senior had made his discovery (which was of course a closely guarded secret) while out walking in the neighbourhood of his home, and it so excited him that he gave up his death-dealing profession and instead founded an enormously up-market stammering school in a local mansion, complete with pedigree herds of cattle and stabling for forty horses. Well-to-do patients brought their own mounts and were provided additionally with concerts and opportunities for amateur theatricals.

Particularly interesting, on account of the legal action it engendered, was the school run by the Hunts, father and son. When the father died in 1851 (his proud claim that he could teach stammerers to read aloud fluently within half an hour wasn't difficult, actually: reading aloud is

[1] See Appendix 1.

usually the least of a stammerer's difficulties) the school property was taken over by his landlord, a dealer in children's clothes. This man kept the school going on his own account: during his regular rent-collecting visits he had seemingly gleaned enough of the secret Hunt 'method' to be able to continue it with no assistance from Hunt's son James. Sustained litigation was necessary by Hunt Junior before the method could be established as its originator's property, handed down legally now to James, and therefore not available for the use of an opportunist ex-children's clothes dealer. The issue, in short, was one of copyright.

Copyright concerns continued, however, and the pirating of secret treatments. As late as the 1880s one school proprietor was so possessive of his secret method that he placed all his patients under a one hundred pound bond against its disclosure.

In the Hunt case, interestingly, no record exists of any dissatisfied patients during the usurped rule of the children's clothes dealer. In fact the man must have done a pretty good job, for the reputation of the school remained unsullied, and once the dealer was ousted James could return. He ran his father's enterprise successfully for many more years, treating over 1,700 patients.

In North America, meanwhile, private enterprise of the devious sort had flourished. In the early 1800s a Dr Yates had established a New York stuttering clinic run by 'the widow Leigh', who was also the governess of his daughter. He too had a secret method, which in fact boiled down to learning to keep the tip of the tongue upon the palate while talking. It's hard to imagine how he prospered, since this is virtually impossible to do, but the challenge must have inspired his patients, for prosper he did. And in due course he was able to sell his 'secret' for a large sum to a Monsieur Malebouche (surely a pseudonym) who then sold it on, for an even larger sum, to the Prussian and Belgian governments. They then farmed it out, untested, to three other doctors who applied it, to their own considerable financial advantage, throughout Europe. They had a good run for their money, for it wasn't until 1828 that the French Academy of Sciences finally exposed the 'Yates method' as useless and its practitioners as charlatans.

The nineteenth century was a great time for quack remedies. Medicine was an increasingly respectable and well-trained profession, but even the growing number of skilled practitioners couldn't possibly keep pace with the needs of a hypochondriac and gullible population (they still can't). So there was money to be made, both by the unscrupulous hands-on operator and – as the files of the London patent office show – by the well-meaning, mechanically minded amateur inventor.

In 1884 the London Hospital for Affections of Speech was founded, with 850 out-patients in its first year. In 1911 this was complemented by a speech clinic at St Bartholomew's, and six years later a speech research centre was established in the West End Hospital for Nervous Diseases. Its head, Dr G. W. Scripture, published a book in which remarkably he recommended treatments along Freudian, psychoanalytical lines. Years ahead of its time, this is a powerful and very sympathetic treatise: among the case histories Dr Scripture quotes is a boy so distressed by his stammer that he flings himself down upon the floor and asks his mother how he can die. Another stammerer, a young woman, presents herself in his consulting room demanding to be either cured or chloroformed. Books like this, although intended for the profession and presumably little read by the general public, must have contributed greatly to the gradual change in popular attitudes towards stammering that took place around this time.

Among medical men, certainly, the twentieth century clearly brought a different, gentler approach. Their writings became much less hortatory. There's little talk of careless habits, idleness, attention-getting, dissipation, life-sapping masturbation: the emphasis is on psychoneuroses, or 'nervous dread', and treatments feature support rather than bracing exhortations. It was a Dr Grierson, for example, who in 1901 first floated the notion that an ex-stammerer makes the best therapist, since only he truly understands the patient's agonies. This idea was particularly eagerly espoused in the United States, where several of the most distinguished writers and therapists of the 1930s, 1940s and 1950s would be ex-stammerers.

In general, the nineteenth century's approach to stammering was typically mechanistic, characterised by an interest in *what* was wrong, while twentieth-century medical men concerned themselves more with *why* it was wrong. Indeed, by 1931 London County Council speech clinics had thrown the baby out with the bath-water and were abjuring all speech re-education as dangerous interference, claiming that in all but the very slightest cases the services of a trained psychiatrist were essential.

Which is not to say that old-school elocutionists weren't still around. There's always a market for traditional methods, no matter how loony. Accordingly the Rev J. Edgar Foster – a reassuringly patrician monicker if ever I heard one – was offering to cure impediments of speech for a guinea a lesson at his Kensington School of Elocution, while a few years earlier a 'Speech Correction School' up in Accrington proposed to cure stammering by substituting the patient's 'natural voice' with a 'new voice' – they cited the example of the famous writer and clergyman Charles Kingsley, whose considerable stammer was widely known to disappear when he mounted the pulpit steps and assumed his preaching manner. The Speech Correction School's literature is unusually confident, even for the period: 'Remember you are following a certainty; correct your voice and your stammer will leave you.'

Down in London, after the Great War, the drama teacher Elsie Fogarty set about improving what she called her patients' 'faulty breathing'. Other post-war elocutionists clung to Victorian moralistic notions and instituted bans on vices such as drinking and smoking, as well as the fairly conventional (and for stammerers totally impossible) remedy of 'relaxation of the face muscles'.

By the 1930s, particularly in America, mainstream medical men had completely abandoned all ideas of blame, or even of patient responsibility. Indeed, with relation to stammering children, the affliction was considered diagnosogenic – that is, it didn't exist until the interference of a diagnostician created it. Not only was this an attractive proposition but for a while the evidence seemed to support it. Some of the evidence, that is – the disfluencies of many children do in reality go away if nobody takes any notice of them – but unfortunately not all.

In adults, psychotherapy was widely undertaken, and if

causes were looked for, it was the stammerer's parents who came under the most suspicion. This was the heyday of psychiatry's great unload-everything-onto-your-parents movement. There were inevitably dissident voices, and they gained ground steadily. Even so, it took a pretty monstrous foghorn of a therapist to proclaim, in 1971, that 'the complexities that have bedevilled the stammering situation since the beginning of the century arise mainly from the introduction of experimental psychotherapy'. But then, these words appeared in the introduction to *his* very mechanistic self-help manual, full of breathing exercises and sitting up straight and paying attention, in which he also wrote, equally arrogantly, 'The only likelihood of failure (after reading this book) lies in a half-hearted attitude on the part of the stammerer.'

I am reminded of another dangerously confident British therapist a few years earlier, in 1950, who wrote: 'The doctor *knows*, let us make no mistake about it, he *knows* how *normal* speech is achieved.' (The italics are his.) Maybe they had the courage of their ignorance back in those days. I can't imagine any doctor today being willing to claim that he knew how anything as complex and mysterious as 'normal' speech (whatever that may be) is achieved.

After the Second World War, the problems of the stammerer were sufficiently widely recognised by officialdom in Britain for the new Labour government to pass legislation obliging local authorities to provide special education for a fairly wide category of children they described as 'verbally impaired'. The Act has been amended, most significantly in 1981, but in spite of this it still contains a loophole: it doesn't specify exactly which local government department is to be responsible for fulfilling this obligation, and so allows wriggling space for shifty, penny-pinching, Treasury-ridden local bureaucrats. Pin down an administrator today and you'll always find that the shortfall you're complaining about is the fault of the other fellow's department.

Adult stammerers received public sympathy also – perhaps partly as a result of the nation's conscience being sharpened by the many trauma-induced speech impediments the war produced – and in 1945 the College of Speech Therapists was founded in London, to legitimise and monitor the profession – or, as one founder member forcefully put it, to protect the public from 'the crass stupidities of the type of disappointed pupil at an elocution school who, when she realises she is not destined for Hollywood stardom, turns reluctantly to speech therapy'. The progress towards social acceptance that stammering made during this period may also be due to King George VI's courageous and very public struggles with his stammer in his speeches and radio broadcasts: these touched the hearts of his subjects and so may have warmed them basically towards the affliction. Certainly the King's example cheered up those stammerers who, like me, grew up in his reign.

In the post-war years stammering's progress away from being mostly an occasion for ridicule, for children's teasing and adults' sniggers, as that of other mental and physical handicaps, has continued and accelerated. This progress has been spearheaded by organisations like Britain's Association For Stammerers (AFS), which is a member of the European League of Stuttering Associations (in 1991 ELSA received direct funding from the European Commission), and by other support groups such as the Plus Club in Sweden, which provide liaison, a sort of national debating society, between self-help groups and professional therapists. In North America the US National Council of Adult Stutterers, founded back in 1966, works with the National Stuttering Project, and seeks, in its literature's touching words, 'to make stutterers proud – not that they stutter, for only a fool can take pride in infirmity – but that they are doing something to help themselves'.

Behind all this there's always the risk of getting over-earnest. Like most other afflictions, stammering has its lighter side, and it would be foolish to pretend otherwise. In the 1920s a British comic actor, Askew Sothern, enjoyed enormous theatrical success both here and in the United States with his portrayal of one Lord Dundreary, a seedy aristocrat whose principal amusing feature seems to have been his stammer. Before him, in 1894, there was a very popular comic novel featuring 'Stuttering Sam – the Whitest Sport of Santa Fe', while a few years before that Smetana had presented a comic stuttering simpleton in his opera *The Bartered Bride*. Stammers in fiction are usually amusing. Not so Dante's 'stuttering crone, squint-eyed, club-footed, both her hands deformed, and her complexion like a white-washed stone . . .' With everything else that was wrong with her, I can't really see why she needed a stutter, but there you are.

Should stammerers mind when unfriendly stereotypes are reinforced like this? At the risk of sounding solemn, I think we should. Apart from anything else, there are knock-on effects. These aren't always obvious, and they can start very young. A therapist recently reported this from one of her young patients: 'My sisters say girls don't do these things. My parents think it's wrong too. I can tell from the way they look at me – like I'm a freak or something . . .'

Even so, sensitivity can be overdone, especially when it's institutionalised. So I was glad to read a recent letter in the British press from the director of the AFS, repudiating protests made by the National Stuttering Project in the United States against scenes in the John Cleese film *A Fish Called Wanda*, in which the character played by Michael Palin is made fun of because of his stammer. Although the film is clearly sympathetic towards Palin's character, the protests were so successful that the film's US distributors cut the scenes altogether. The AFS disagrees: 'The great majority of our members want more openness and less embarrassment about stammering, so that they do not have to hide their affliction. The last thing they want is 'politically correct' censorship.'

I agree. Just as I agree with the AFS's intervention when another recent film, *Dead Again*, gave the clear impression that stammering could be cured by hypnosis. Since this isn't true and might easily give a lot of people false hope, the AFS was quick to express its concern publicly – which the film's star, Frankie Howerd, a stammerer himself, readily supported. It's a question of choosing your cases.

To do justice to the work of national stammering associations, and their history, would fill several chapters. As far as the British AFS is concerned, I believe its quarterly newsletter alone is worth the small membership fee, not to mention its many other activities: its watchdog role, its workshops, specialist advice leaflets, local self-help group directory, library, information service . . . the list goes on. Anybody who stammers or is involved in the life of a stammerer should join. Significantly, when the AFS recently gained brief coverage on a breakfast television show, more than three hundred serious enquiries were received at its headquarters within the next two days.

Many of these enquiries concerned stammering 'schools'. These are still around, although the length of the residential courses available is much shorter than those generally offered in the last century. We don't know precisely what went on in Victorian stammering schools: mostly various forms of rhythmic speech seem to have been taught, often to the accompaniment of strenuous callisthenics; group reading aloud in unison was practised, and there was dire emphasis on discipline, early rising, cold showers and *esprit de corps* – as in the public school system at large. Three months of this seems to have been the average course duration.

Such methods persisted well into the twentieth century. The American therapist Charles Van Riper has written revealingly of one such school that he himself attended in the 1920s. His stay began with two weeks of total silence, rigorously enforced. If pupils transgressed, more days were added to their sentence. The boys were kept half-starved in Spartan boarding houses, and good behaviour (i.e. stammer-free sentences) was rewarded with extra beans or tokens cashable at the school tuck shop. The 'treatment' consisted principally of swinging Indian clubs for hours on end to improve lung capacity, chanting in unison, and inspirational harangues from the school principal. Van Riper says it was only his desperate need to believe that persuaded him to submit.

Any pupil who expressed doubt about the Method was instantly expelled, and the head teacher then lectured the remaining boys on his ruined life, his sad future, his blighted hopes of happiness and prosperity. Outside speakers in expensive clothes visited every week, claiming to be ex-pupils of the school, and described their successful cures.

Van Riper suspects that these men must have been fraudulent, hired by the principal. Certainly, of the sixty-five boys from his intake to whom he wrote afterwards, only one claimed to have profited from the treatment. Although all of them had been fluent by the end of the course, and had signed testimonials to that effect, within six months most were worse than they'd been at the start. Van Riper followed up on the boy claiming to have been cured, spoke to him, and found that although he spoke without stammering, it was at a regular two syllables per second, like a zombie, so that it was almost impossible to understand him. Van Riper himself gained no help at all from the course.

Today's residential courses are less punitive in their approach, and of shorter duration, most lasting a week or a fortnight. A typical course seems to cost around £500 (as of May 1992), exclusive of accommodation. Numbers of patients are small, eight to ten, and the treatment is intensive, using the latest techniques and technology, together with counselling in self-image and preparedness for change.

Also on the market today are various mechanical aids and appliances for the stammerer that are equal in their ingenuity to anything produced by the Victorians. In Japan there are many finely crafted in-mouth devices, such as celluloid strips worn behind the teeth and whistles to fit beneath the tongue that are so delicately tuned that only the user can hear them when they sound their warnings of faulty speech production. In Europe more expensive gadgets are marketed, varieties of metronome either for the breast pocket or to hook behind the ear, as well as little stingers designed to prick or, with a small electric shock, otherwise jolt the stammerer out of his block. There's also a small, very hi-tech packet of electronics that delivers a version of the stammerer's speech, delayed by a few thousandths of a second, to his ears by means of headphones and to his neck in the region of his vocal cords by means of a discreet vibrator. The promotional leaflet warns that the headphones are for use 'only in a clinical setting or in the privacy of your home or office'. I'm glad to hear that vibrating in public is out.

Therapeutic techniques are wide-ranging. Stammers seem to get better when the stammerer can't hear his own voice, and there's a buzzer called the Edinburgh Masker that does the job: in Russia a similar device was the Derazne Correctophone. On a less sophisticated level, back in 1965 ice cream was found to be an effective remedy when administered liberally to one lucky American lad every time he didn't stammer.

My own favourite therapy is culled from the reader's letter in a recent edition of the AFS magazine: 'To correct our habit . . . he'd just hit us as soon as we got stuck over a sentence. Really hard, too. It went on from 6 am until 9 pm and was the most revolting course you could imagine. But in three days we were all cured, and I've never stammered since.'

Finally, before all British speech therapists equip themselves with knuckledusters, they should be reminded what an extremely idiosyncratic business curing a stammer seems to be. I'm not sure what they should learn from it, but there's a well-attested case of a 1950s stammerer who reported a total cure after eating the meat of a black tomcat at midnight under a half moon, and drinking the urine from a virgin mare.

It will be clear by now that I'm avoiding any serious comment here on the effectiveness of any of these techniques, courses or appliances, past or present. Treatments for stammering are a complex, controversial subject, and I'll be giving them a chapter of their own later.

Meanwhile, what does this brief history of stammering tell us? First, that no stammerer need feel alone or a freak: he's a member of a large, ancient, and often distinguished company – he's maybe one in a hundred, which is roughly the percentage of the population with rhesus negative blood, and *they're* not considered freaks. And second, that the prevalence of stammering is hardly surprising. Speech is a recent human acquisition and might be said to be still in the prototype stage. It's a perilous business. Maybe evolution hasn't ironed out all the wrinkles yet.

As two thoughtful speech researchers, Walls and Myers, put it in 1986: 'That language development is an enormous undertaking during childhood cannot be denied. Phonological, syntactic, semantic and pragmatic developments are all occurring at a feverish pace during the very period that the speech production system is maturing. These variables interact increasingly as the child matures, during those critical early years of development.'

It's hardly surprising, then, that the process sometimes goes wrong.

~

Patrick Campbell was a brilliant journalist and television personality. I vividly remember reading his pieces about his stammer when I was growing up, back in the 1940s. They encouraged me a lot. They were also very funny.

The story below is much quoted, but I make no apology for that. It's a classic.

From my earliest days I have enjoyed an attractive impediment in my speech. I have never permitted the use of the word 'stammer'. I can't say it myself. This surprising phenomenon has assumed, in its time, a wide variety of different forms, and the ability to change its nature without warning. For instance, I used to have for several weeks at a time what I came to call the 'muted gibbon' cry. It used to go, 'May I awah awah awash my ahah ahah ahah ahah ahands please?'

At a formal dinner party, a particularly dynamic form of this stammer made its debut. At this time I was having the muted gibbon call, with rotation. That is, my head turned ponderously from right to left, and then back again, with the effort of speech. It humped the muscles of my neck like a bison and, in fact, rendered any attempt at articulation completely out of the question.

But I threw myself into it. I set myself to say, 'I went bathing yesterday and the water was as warm as toast.' I became locked at once. My head turned slowly to the left, the rich blood already pounding into my face. I met the terrified gaze of the diplomat's wife, tried to smile at her, emitted three 'ahah ahah ahah's' instead, and then found myself centred upon Theodore (another stammerer, but one who prefaced his attempted speech with a whistle), immediately opposite me. To my absolute consternation I saw that he was busy too. The fool had thrown himself into speech as well, and was now whistling away in short, piercing trills, with his eyes clamped firmly shut. My head ground round to the right. 'I awah awah awent . . .' I said to the brisk matron, and then my head started its journey back again. I caught a glimpse of Mrs Gilbert out of the corner of my eye. Her lips were moving in prayer. I had time to think that she was lucky to have them moving at all, when I became based upon Theodore once more. He must have played the whole of *The Bluebells of Scotland* by this time, but was as far away as ever from saying anything.

It went on through all eternity, some of the guests leaning forward with bright smiles and the perspiration running down their faces, others suddenly exhibiting nervous mannerisms of their own, twitching or plucking at their clothes, or coughing loudly, but all waiting to hear what either Theo or I might have to add to the fund of human knowledge.

Mrs Gilbert broke down in the end. Her voice, when she found it, came out in a scream, but she managed to speak. The guests leaped in their seats as if shot, but she'd done it. In another moment the whole lot of them were chattering away again – high-pitched nervous stuff, but at least it was coming out. Theodore and I let ourselves unwind slowly, and the rest of the dinner played itself out without incident.

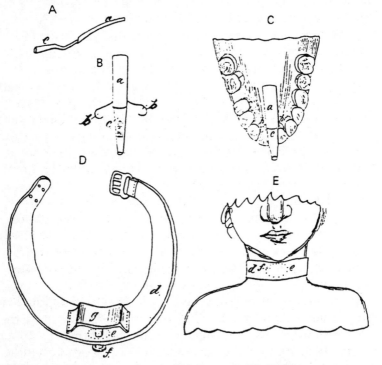

FIGURE 1.5 The Bates appliances. (U.S. Patent 8, 394 [1851].)

3

What is a stammer? What is a cure?

. . . my name is more or less Donald . . .

It seems clear enough. A 'stammer', a 'cure for a stammer' . . . we talk about them all the time – surely it would take a really dedicated expert to make an issue out of defining either? Either a man has a stammer or he hasn't, either it's cured or it isn't, and you don't need a degree from the College of Speech and Language Therapists to be able to spot the difference.

Unfortunately life isn't that easy. Genuine difficulties lie in wait; genuine obstacles to the simple answer.

The first, most obvious difficulty is created by the important distinction we make between the verb 'to stammer' (neutral, a behaviour), and the noun 'a stammerer' (judgmental, a deviant). Our subtle appreciation of this distinction is shown in remarks like, 'He doesn't stammer enough to be called a stammerer.' Or sometimes, 'He's not really a stammerer – he only stammers because he can't always find the word he wants.' It doesn't matter if this is a fair distinction or not – it betrays our confusion. A stammer is both a single event, which we excuse, and a series of events, which we don't. (I use *excuse* here in the sense of *overlook*, but there is in fact often an element of blame around in our reaction, even today.)

But in any case, we were looking for a simple definition, and already questions of judgment are creeping in.

Secondly, we have to examine our widely shared perception of stammering as a speech defect. In reality, ninety-nine per cent of stammerers do not have a speech defect. They can speak perfectly well. They often do. Stammering actors declaim unhesitatingly on the stage, solitary stammerers chat in a comradely fashion with their dogs, stammering parsons are all too fluent in the pulpit. The stammerer's difficulty isn't primarily with his speech, it's with his relationship to his audience. It isn't a speech defect, it's a communication defect.

Maybe that sounds picky, but it's true. The importance of the audience relationship is best demonstrated by the results of a lengthy series of experiments in reading aloud to different audiences that were carried out back in the 1950s. And not even reading aloud to real people – the experiment was fined down till stammerers were reading aloud to *photographs* of people. The tests showed conclusively that subjects stammered more when their reading was addressed to a photograph of a 'hard' person (an authority figure, a headmaster or a parent) than when it was to a photograph of a 'soft' person (a child or a friend). In short, the subtle relationship a stammerer has with his audience influences his speech even if that audience is no more than a symbol, an idea, a shiny black-and-white photograph.

This may seem ridiculous – certainly it's hard to credit – but it's a fact, and the conclusion to be drawn from it is inescapable. Stammerers are able to talk, and to read aloud, perfectly well. There's nothing wrong with the physical mechanisms of their speech: the basic difficulty isn't to do with muscles, phonation, respiration, articulation, it's to do with confidence, control and identity.

In terms of a definition, though, does all this matter? As one famous American expert famously said, 'Everyone but the expert knows what stuttering is.' So long as there's a vague sort of general consensus on the subject (which of course there is), aren't all these arguments about basic difficulties, and whether we're judgmental or not, really just a quibble?

I don't think so. Definitions don't come on their own. They're not the last word on any subject: they have implications. And they're circular: they tend to grow out of attitudes, and from then on to form them. For example, there are therapists who have liked to define stammering as what a man does when he's trying not to stammer. Now that's clever stuff, very neat, very droll, but it grows out of the belief that once he stops trying not to stammer he'll no longer need to, and it passes that belief on . . . with profound implications for the conduct of future therapy. Now this may be a good thing and it may be a bad, and this isn't the chapter for discussing therapies. The point is, definitions have to be just right, for they cast long shadows.

After all, most people are familiar with the openly judgmental definitions of stammering – it's just a bad habit, it's just wanting to draw attention to yourself, it's just not thinking before you talk – and are aware of the impatient, bullying responses they produce. On the other hand, although no adverse judgments are involved, when people believe a stammer, like a limp or myopia, to be the result of some physical defect, their mistake is still dangerous for it leads them to expect consistency, and then sooner or later to the familiar, irritated, hurtful comment, 'You should see him with his friends – he can talk perfectly well when he wants to.'

When he wants to . . . Dear God, when *doesn't* he want to?

The purpose of a correct definition is to help people get things right. Not the way they want things to be, and not the way we or anybody else want them to be, but *right* . . . And for a definition to do that it needs to be simple, well-informed, accurate, and as objective as anything human can ever be.

So what exactly is a stammer? We've already encountered a couple of obstacles in the way of a simple, well-informed, accurate and objective definition, and now there's a third: a difficulty in differentiating a stammer from the 'normal' disfluencies that nice ordinary people get up to. Many therapists claim that there's very little a stammerer does that is different from the *ums* and *ers* and *y'knows* and syllable repetitions that are a part of most non-stammerers' speech. Often these, especially the repetitions, are virtually indistinguishable from a stammerer's disfluencies.

Certainly this is a very important point to remember when considering the speech of young children. Most of the disfluencies that young children produce are entirely normal. But stammering in children is a very special subject, and I'll just emphasise here that diagnosis should never be rushed.

Be suspicious of anyone, friend, relative or expert, who offers a quick opinion.

As far as adult stammerers are concerned, I'm worried when I hear therapists point out the similarities between the disfluencies of stammerers and those of non-stammerers. I realise that this is intended to make their patients feel better about their own speech and therefore about themselves. But it brings with it the implication that they really aren't all that different from non-stammerers – with the further implication that change won't really be all that difficult. And I'm worried because I believe there's a false assumption at work. Like isn't being compared with like. I believe that the fluent speaker's *ums* and *ers* and careless repetitions are fundamentally different from the spasms and muscular disruptions that the stammerer battles with. The *ums* are friendly filler noises, put in to make talking easier. The stammerer's spasms are hostile interruptions: they're forced on him and they make talking unimaginably harder.

In the best of all possible worlds the therapist would always know best. But this isn't the best of all possible worlds, and I know I'm not dangerously undermining the medical profession when I suggest that now and then a therapist is just slightly less than infallible. And in the matter of fluent speech *vis-à-vis* disfluent I do not believe that – as some of her kind propose – there is a smooth continuum from total fluency across to severe stammering, with most people occupying a position somewhere in the middle. I believe there are two different and quite separate phenomena. There is normal speech, with a continuum from very fluent to very disfluent, and there is stammering speech, with a similar continuum from very fluent to very disfluent. Thus it's possible that a normal speaker at the disfluent end of his continuum may be less coherent than a stammerer at the fluent end of his – but the non-stammerer's incoherence is of a different order from the stammerer's. One is surface stuff. The other is gut-wrenching.

I admit that to the outsider they may sound very much the same. I also admit that, to complicate matters, experienced stammerers stick in normal-sounding *ums* and *ers* and *y'knows* on purpose, to disguise the true nature of their problem. So pity the poor therapist.

Before she can decide upon a treatment, or even that one's necessary, she has to arrive at a diagnosis. Before she can arrive at a diagnosis she has to make an assessment. Before she can make an assessment she has to have a definition of what she's assessing. And the simple, well-informed, accurate, objective definition that we're all looking for has so far eluded us.

When is a stammer not a stammer?
When it's a normal disfluency.
How can we tell the difference?
By asking the stammerer.
That's not very objective. I thought we were trying to be objective.
Why don't you jump off a roof or something?
When faced with this awkward sort of problem, the sensible thing for any professional to do is to side-step it; to look instead for something that *does* respond to the analytical method, and then to devise a system for quantifying it, rating it according to some objective standard. Speech therapists home in on the assessment stage. They may not be able to define what it is they're assessing but they can sure as hell have a go at breaking it down into its components, into 'stammering episodes', and then devise a system for quantifying them, rating them for frequency and mean duration.

To do this they use a video recorder and a stop-watch. The theory now is that if a patient produces fewer, or shorter, 'stammering episodes' over a given number of syllables than he did the previous time he was tested, then presumably he's stammering less. And if this happens after a period of treatment, then the therapist may fairly hope that it is at least in part because of the treatment. So she's doing something right.

There's an obvious weakness here. The video camera doesn't distinguish between genuine 'stammering episodes' and those instances of normal disfluency we've already discussed. So the science immediately breaks down and we're back with subjective judgments, in this case those of whichever researcher happens to be holding the stop-watch and staring at the video screen: 'Umm . . . that glitch *there* is a genuine stammer, making seven hundred and thirty-two . . . umm . . . no, that one *there* is just a touch of heartburn . . .'

In any case, even when genuine copper-bottomed 'stammering episodes' can be agreed, the relationship between frequency and duration is hard to compare and assess. For example, one report describes a test in which most of the subjects, on a good day, were producing around a hundred blocks or repetitions per five thousand syllables (a fairly average count, incidentally). One subject, however, produced only three blocks, and no repetitions, in his five thousand syllables – but his blocks were of respectively one, two, and three-and-a-quarter minutes in duration . . . The report doesn't tell us how he was rated. What would you say? Count out for yourself a block of just one minute. Personally, I cannot imagine the agony of a stammer that blocked me for three-and-a-quarter minutes. The strain of one such block would be enough to knock out most people for the rest of the day.

In their pursuit of an assessment tool, researchers are prepared to go to impressive lengths. The 1960s invention of electromyography – the ability to record electrical potentials from the muscles – gave them an exciting new technique. By the application of tiny electrodes in exactly the right areas researchers have been able to measure laryngeal activity during stammering, the involvement of the orbicularis, masseter and geniohyoid (the articulatory) muscles, and even to detect 'inappropriate bursts of muscular activity during silence'. So what hope do stammerers have if they stammer when they're not even speaking?

Also, by the use of fibre optics, they've been able to observe the glottis during stammering, and the condition of the vocal folds. Other clever devices have enabled them to measure aerodynamic patterns, intra-oral pressure, and the rate of air-flow from the oral cavity during speech. The breakthrough here is that 'multiple elevations of intra-oral pressure without air-flow' have been detected during their patients' silent blocks. If they'd asked me I could have told them that, and much more cheaply. We strain, but nothing bloody well comes out.

If I seem to be taking this work less than seriously, that's truly not out of any wish to devalue it. Nobody knows of what genuine clinical interest and use such findings may one day be. It's just that I'm boggling at the mental picture it gives me: teams of volunteer stammerers, wired for sound, fibre optic tubes down their throats, electrodes dotting their tongues, their faces festooned with cables, their oral cavities stuffed with wind-speech indicators, their laboratory couches surrounded with computer screens. And in spite of all this they're still stammering doggedly on. I'd have expected the whole performance to put them off speaking, if not stammering, for life.

And there are yet more tests to come. Stammerers typically have higher-than-average blood pressure and pulse rate: these will have to be confirmed. Their brains have unusual alpha waves, and these too will have to be studied, by means of electroencephalograph recordings. Then there's their interesting binocular inco-ordination, otherwise known as *temporary strabismus* . . .

I love that *temporary strabismus*. I'm not sure why, but it puts me in mind of magnificent central-European consulting rooms with walnut panelling and horse-hair sofas. Paraphrasing Yeats, I'd rather have *temporary strabismus* than be Lord of Upper Egypt.

But all this brings us no nearer to a simple, well-informed, accurate, objective definition of stammering.

The fact is, there doesn't seem to be one. At the lengthy end of the wordage scale there's the catch-all definition favoured by Britain's College of Speech and Language Therapists: the college defines stammering as 'Speech characterised by interruptions in its fluency by the repetition of sounds, syllables or phrases, and blocks, overt or disguised, often accompanied by concomitant movements and disruption of normal breathing rhythm. There may be avoidance reactions either of words or of speech situations.'

This is the scattershot approach, and at first sight it doesn't seem to let much get away. But one has to be troubled by the weasel phrase 'overt or disguised'. Overt blocks are easy enough to spot, but if a block isn't overt, how does one tell if it's 'disguised' or simply isn't there? Then again, no distinction is made between stammered repetitions and 'normal' repetitions, and there's no mention at all of the quality that has to be stammering's most unmistakable feature, its compulsiveness, its perseveration in the face of everything the poor bloody stammerer throws at it.

At the other end of the wordage scale there's an admirably no-nonsense definition offered by the respected American speech therapist, Oliver Bloodstein. Dr Bloodstein bluntly defines the disorder as 'Whatever is perceived as stuttering by a reliable observer who has relatively good agreement with others.'

Brief and to the point. All the same, what with 'reliable observer', and 'relatively good agreement', it's clear that the good doctor doesn't rate objectivity or accuracy all that highly. He leaves us with the advice that a man either stammers or doesn't stammer, and you only need to be a 'reliable observer' to be able to spot the difference. And that is the proposition I put forward at the beginning of this chapter. So it looks as if I've taken you three times round the shrubbery and got you back where you started.

Maybe I have. But I've aired some probably unfamiliar aspects of the problem on the way, and I've also put forward a couple of official solutions.

There's a third contender. One that's both the best and the worst. It's the best because it does the job, and it's the worst because it's an acronym and everybody hates acronyms. In the introductory chapter of this book I mentioned the letters CPSDS, and explained that they stood for Chronic Perseverative Speech Disfluency Syndrome. Well, CPSDS may indeed be revolting jargon, but it's simple, well-informed, accurate and objective. And it's also economical. Just five words, each of which makes a vital contribution:

> *Chronic* we know about: it's a fair description.
>
> *Perseverative* covers stammering's very important compulsiveness.
>
> *Speech Disfluency* summarises all the word-oriented difficulties.
>
> *Syndrome* embraces not only the head jerks and eye rollings but also the physiological symptoms, everything from the condition of the vocal folds to dear old *temporary strabismus*.

If I were a purist, then, I'd vote for CPSDS. It defines all the significant features of a stammer in the shortest possible span. But unfortunately there's one further requirement for a definition. As well as being simple, well-informed, accurate, objective and economical, it needs to be user friendly.

And CPSDS, even in its full form *Chronic Perseverative Speech Disfluency Syndrome* (perhaps especially in its full form), is a total turn-off. Eyes glaze. Cheeks pale. Feet fidget. I do not lie, I've seen them.

Having taken you within sight of the Promised Land, therefore, I shall drag you back, seek refuge in common sense, and settle for Dr Bloodstein. For the purposes of this book, and of anything else you care to think of, a stammer is 'Whatever is perceived as such by a reliable observer who has relatively good agreement with others.'

All he really fails on is objectivity which these days scientists will tell us is all an illusion, anyway.

An apology's due. I find I've been guilty of a bad case of putting the cart before the horse. I've spent all this time defining stammering in terms of its symptoms but I haven't yet got round to agreeing just what those symptoms are. And once we've decided to use Dr Bloodstein's 'reliable observer' as our stammer definer it's particularly important to establish sound criteria for that observer to work with. So bear with me while I backtrack.

First, there's the basic team of stammer symptoms everybody knows. Its most obvious members are: blocks and repetitions. Blocks are those moments when the entire speech mechanism fuses solid, when the stammer snake wraps himself tightly round the whole outfit and hangs on. They're moments of faint gasping (aaarghh), or of total silence (. . .), during which the stammerer labours and nothing emerges.

Repetitions are the opposite of these. The snake's feeling skittish, the stammerer labours, and all too much emerges; mostly obnoxious numbers of the word's initial letter (p-p-p-penguin), or of its initial syllable (tay-tay-tay-table). The middles of words get blocked or repeated also (disgus-gus-gus-gusting), but less commonly.

These front-line symptoms are usually accompanied by other activities; gratuitous thoughtful frowns, tapping feet, attempts to distract the listener's attention by gesturing vigorously out of the window. These may once have been conscious devices – not symptoms at all, but ways of dealing with or disguising symptoms – and they may even once have worked. But by the time the stammerer has lived with his affliction for a year or two, they'll have lost whatever ability they ever had to make things easier for him and they'll just be hangers-on, members of the symptom team with two left feet.

Other team members are craftier – they too aim to make life easier for the stammerer, but they do it less noticeably, either by postponing crises or by avoiding them. Word post-ponements usually take the form of interjected phrases, intended to give the stammerer a chance to step back and take a run at whatever's bothering him. These tend either to be superfluous ('It's g-g-g- . . . I do believe it might be going to rain'), or just plain silly ('My name is D-D-D- . . . my name is more or less Donald'). Word avoidances mostly employ substitutions ('I'm going to catch a b-b-b- . . . one of those public transport things'), or last-minute changes of mind ('Thank you, I'd love a cup of t-t-t- . . . of coffee').

As well as word avoidances there are situation avoidances. As far as the stammerer is concerned these have a one hun-dred per cent success rate (who's troubled by his stammer when he's at home in bed, with his head under the blankets?), but they don't do much for his social or pro-fessional prospects.

Other team members may be pipe stems to chomp on, assumed funny voices or heavy foreign accents, anything at all that distracts the stammer snake from going about its business.

It's a big squad, and every stammerer puts together his own. Most of its members will be played out, of no functional value – they scored once but they're old now and the oppo-sition runs rings round them – but their team manager keeps them on the payroll, maybe for old times' sake. The players a stammerer fields on any given night may vary, but he rarely pensions any off.

The best of the bunch are undoubtedly the word avoid-ances. They actually do quite often work: the stammerer has words or sounds that he knows from experience are likely to give him hell, so he scans ahead and tries to dodge round them. He's often wrong – on some days his stammer snake will leap up and grab at the easiest words while letting old enemies go by with its blessing – but he's right often enough to make it worth the effort. There's one thing he learns early on: nothing's certain in his life, not even d-d-death or t-t-taxes.

Certainly listeners can be expected to give him difficulty too. Bus conductors in a hurry. Telephone operators, whether in a hurry or not. People who ask him his name, people who ask him the way to the nearest bus stop – he knows that too but he seldom gets past the first word. And there are always those photographs of bosses or headmasters . . . Unlike word avoidances, listener avoidances aren't all that easy. There are people he just *has* to talk to. For my part, to her dying day I don't believe my poor mother heard a single fluent sentence.

One characteristic symptom that all stammers share is their variability. They change constantly; from day to day and from moment to moment; from listener to listener; from situation to situation; from subject to subject; from cloud in the sky to cloud in the sky. Patterns may be observed, but they're never reliable. Maybe there's a man who finds intimate subjects 'difficult' – pimples or bowel movements – yet the same man will be able to describe his sexual goings-on with distressing fluency. 'Easy' days may be associated with the stammerer's general well-being – women find that their stammers fluctuate with their menstrual cycles – yet every stammerer has had moments of carefree abandon that are unexpectedly shattered by verbal catatonia.

There will be 'easy' situations too. Inconveniently, one of the easiest is often the speech clinic. Therapists fairly complain that they often have to treat disorders they themselves scarcely ever see. Particularly if they've been successful in establishing themselves as 'easy' listeners. A therapist's life is seldom simple.

Not that any outsider can safely predict who an 'easy' listener will be. A person you know? A person you trust? A person you love? Not necessarily. Beloved children and wives often have a dreadful time of it. Then again, one beautifully spoken man I talked to at an AFS meeting explained that he was fluent with me only because I was a total stranger. If he got to know me better, he told me sadly, his stammer would become more and more revolting.

One thing can be said in favour of all this hassle: it makes the stammerer extraordinarily flexible. He has an undemanding attitude to life. He can't afford to be fussy. He takes his pleasures where he can. One man tells me, 'I buy the brand of cigarettes I can say that day.' Another plans his holidays on the basis of places with unthreatening initial letters – he says he's had some pleasant surprises.

Predictably, with all this activity out on the field, there's kibitzing behind the scenes as well. Lots more symptoms, this time physiological, associated with the autonomic system. Sweaty palms are common. Blood sugar rises, so does the adrenalin content in urine. Blood pressure goes up, of course, and pulse rate too. And there's that unusual eye movement, and that unusual alpha wave pattern in the brain.

All this sounds pretty drastic. One wonders how the poor bloody stammerer survives. But there's good news too. Nice ordinary people show exactly the same physiological symptoms . . . if they're excited, or tense, or cross, or frustrated. In short, these symptoms are the normal reaction of any body to its owner being buggered about. And you show me a stammerer who *isn't* excited, tense, cross, frustrated, buggered about – and usually all at the same time.

So stammering's physiological symptoms probably don't much signify. Everybody has them, and for the same reasons. Stammerers have them more, that's all.

There's a symptom I've left to last. It's the ugly one. It's the embarrassing one. But I wouldn't be doing my job here if I let all my jovial anecdotes obscure it. For this is the symptom in which all the others probably find their beginnings, and it's certainly where they all end. In fear. Fear . . . sometimes nagging, often acute. A pain. Fear. Not simply of the stupid daily business of talking. Fear of people. Fear of the world. Fear of life.

At his most vulnerable moment, his most necessary point of contact with his fellow human beings, at his reaching out towards them in speech, be it mundane or intimate, at such times the stammerer may expect to be wounded, made ridiculous, betrayed, destroyed. It's not surprising that one of them has written, 'You take your fear to bed with you, it greets you when you wake up in the morning, and it walks beside you all day.'

This had to be said. It isn't a plea for sympathy. Most

stammerers learn to cope. We're a cheerful lot. Many of us learn to cope very well indeed.

Indeed, in an interview the poet Philip Larkin gave to the *Spectator*, he says, 'And then there was the stammer. Oxford terrified me . . . I still stammered quite badly up to the age of maybe thirty. I mean stammering to the point of handing over little slips of paper at the railway station saying third class to Birmingham, instead of actually trying to get it out. Still, *I soon had several circles of friends* at Oxford. [The italics are mine.] The college circle, the jazz circle, possibly the literary circle . . .'

Larkin isn't asking for sympathy. He coped. *I soon had several circles of friends* . . . Like many stammerers, he coped very well. But for honesty's sake this must be said: even those who cope most successfully still admit that they have been shaped by their fear, and that it never entirely leaves them. And for the rest of us, the less impressive twitchers and battlers and garglers, it's a part of our daily lives.

For the very young there's the daily ordeal of the school roll-call, the question in class, the playground cruelty. A few years later there's the job that's literally at stake if the right word can't be said, there's the receptionist who's going to have to hold that smile until her lipstick cracks, there's the first daily ping of the telephone bell that brings the heart into the mouth. Later still there's the father's fear of causing his children humiliation, there's the early daily planning session as the hours ahead are scanned for crisis points, there's the understanding wife . . . the *need* for an understanding wife. And so it goes.

Enough said. This is the symptomatology of a stammer. What it is, how it's experienced, and the baggage it brings with it. We've agreed on a definition, and we've agreed on a description. The Syndrome. The Chronic Perseverative Speech Disfluency Syndrome, or whatever is perceived as such by a reliable observer who has relatively good agreement with others. The snake in the house of our speech. At last we can move on. We know what we mean by it.

Do we know what we mean by a cure for it?

Getting started on what we meant by a stammer wasn't easy. Getting started on what we mean by a cure for it won't be much easier. The first snag is pretty basic: the word itself. *Cure* seems to be technically inappropriate. We've just got through defining a stammer in terms of its symptoms, and in general terms symptoms don't get cured – they get controlled, alleviated, removed or whatever. It's the disorders causing them that get cured. Or not, as the case may be.

At this point a brief side trip to look at causes seems in order. Nothing in any great detail – there's a whole gang of official candidates and I'll be interviewing them properly later – just a quick survey. So I'd like to begin by proposing that we rule out purely physical causes. Not because stammering may not have them, but because purely physical causes don't have to be expressed solely in terms of their symptoms. Cancer is cancer. Influenza is influenza. The things they do to you are something else. Not that psychosomatic elements don't play their part – a stomach ulcer, for one, although relentlessly physical, is notoriously vulnerable to its owner's rages or anxieties – but physical causes classically have a dogged reliability about their effects that stammers notably lack.

But if we rule out purely physical causes and accept that stammering is principally a disorder of the mind rather than of the body, then *cure* is back in business. Disorders of the mind typically are both defined and cured in terms of their effects, of their symptoms. Depression, agoraphobia, kleptomania – in simplistic terms, once the symptoms of these are dealt with, then we justly claim that the disorders themselves have been cured. For what are they but their symptoms? And what is a stammer but a lot of stammering?

Good point. But there's another snag. Stammering has a lifelong, maybe even a congenital quality. Stammerers who no longer stammer tend to think of themselves as ex-stammerers. They don't think of themselves as nice ordinary people – they're ex-stammerers. Some, like the brilliant theatrical director and television presenter, Dr Jonathan Miller, don't even claim the 'ex'. He speaks with daunting fluency, nobody actually hears him stammer, but he still thinks of himself as a stammerer. His fluency, he says, is the product of constant vigilance. By means of ceaseless verbal ducking and weaving, substitutions, paraphrases, the full resources of a large vocabulary, he's driven his stammer underground. The snake's outwitted. But is it 'cured'?

Just as there's no such thing as a cured alcoholic, there's only an alcoholic who isn't drinking alcohol, maybe in an important sense there's no such thing as a cured stammerer – there's only a stammerer who isn't stammering.

Not that any of this metaphysical speculation is much help when a stammerer presents himself at a speech clinic and asks the therapist (they always do) what she thinks the chances are that she'll be able to cure him. So how does she answer?

In this situation every therapist has her own response. Mine, as a layman, would be to remind the patient that it wasn't basically his speech disorder that drove him to the clinic. Plenty of people with speech disorders never arrive in front of therapists, they simply soldier on. And it isn't a question of degree: some stammerers with terrible disorders soldier on while others with relatively mild ones turn up for treatment. No, what drives a stammerer to seek therapy is the *distress* his speech disorder causes him. If his *distress* can be dealt with (either by making his speech completely fluent or, more probably, by improving his speech and therefore his self-estimation), then the patient will be content. It's the whole man, distress and all, who needs to be treated, and if the therapist is successful then it's the whole man who's cured.

It doesn't matter that by any objective judgment the speech disorder may still be present, and perhaps not much better than it was to begin with. In this situation objective judgments don't apply. If the patient's distress has gone away, he's cured.

It doesn't matter either that some other impediment may be so reduced by therapy as to be almost undetectable. If the patient's nature is such that even one tiny daily block is enough to hang over him and sap his confidence, then there's been no cure.

Subjectivity rules. OK? For once, in this if in nothing else, the patient knows best.

Laugh, and the world laughs with you. If the patient's happy with his stammer, then everybody's happy with his stammer.

But before we finally settle on what we mean by a cure for

stammering, one further, more mechanical element needs considering. A time scale. Days and months, months and years, the duration of the effect. Relapses are notoriously common. Achieving miraculous improvements in fluency is seldom difficult, with even the worst stammerer. Making them stick is. A month, six months, nine months . . . most therapists these days like to keep track of their patients for anything up to a year before they'll consider their treatments successful. This doesn't mean that there's any magical significance about a year – relapses can occur even several years later, for no ex-stammerer seems to be completely secure. It simply means that there has to be a cut-off point somewhere, and it's usually set at a year.

I think that's reasonable. No stammerer should consider his hours in therapy wasted if they give him a year's less stressful speaking. A year is a long time.

So this, at last, is what I think we should mean when we talk about a cure for stammering: any outcome of therapy that sends the patient away content, and that lasts for longer than a year.

It's a pretty minimal definition, and I have to say at once that not every therapist or researcher will agree with me. The easy-going Dr Bloodstein, for one, is in this respect much more demanding. 'The subjects' speech must sound natural and spontaneous,' he tells us, '. . . and the subjects must be free from any need to monitor their speech.'

He's right. Easy, fluent speech, not a single block or gargle, no more watchful avoidances or substitutions . . . in the best of all possible worlds that's what we'd all hold out for. But I've already said it: this isn't the best of all possible worlds, it's the world we live in. The real world. And in the real world, all the evidence suggests that if patients set their hopes so high, an awful lot of them will be disappointed. Worse, if therapists tell them the truth about their prospects within the narrow framework of Dr Bloodstein's definition, an awful lot of them will be frightened off. They'll go back home. They won't even try.

And that would be a very great pity.

Nowadays there are therapies that can help virtually every patient. Stammerers should know this. They must never be put off seeking help by the possibility that they won't end up with perfect speech. What *is* perfect speech, anyway? And who cares? Communication, not speech, is the pot of gold at the end of every stammerer's rainbow.

~

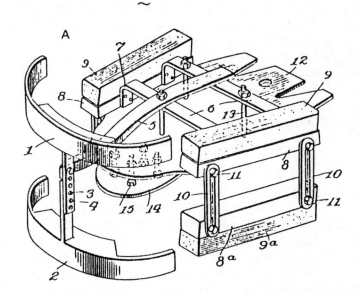

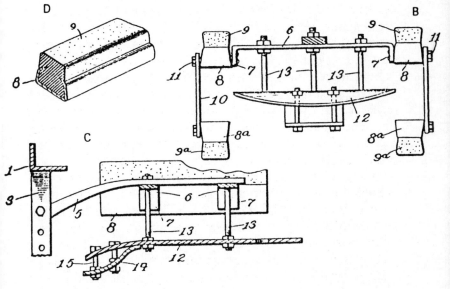

FIGURE 4.3 Beattie and Peake's stammer-cure device to minimize articulation. (British Patent, U.S. Patent 1,030,964 [1912].)

From Letting Go, *the journal of the National Stuttering Project,*
America's equivalent of the British Association for Stammerers.

I really look forward to each issue of *Letting Go* in order
to read the uplifting stories from people who stutter.
People who with great courage find successful solutions
to problems involving stuttering. In addition, some of us
are fortunate enough to belong to National Stuttering Project chapters around the country. At these meetings we
hear optimism voiced by those who stutter as members
tell us of their achievements while encouraging us to do
better . . .

But wait a minute! Why are we always hearing successful stories? Is it because those who write letters or those
who talk at meetings never fail? No, for they claim disappointment and frustration. Yet something about their
manner tells us that they seldom fail.

I had my final chance to rid myself of stuttering in 1974.
My therapy proved successful and although I experienced
some stuttering after that and still called myself a stutterer,
I didn't really stutter much. Other more severe stutterers
looked up to me as one who had made it . . . But in 1982
I started to experience a return to more and more uncon-
trolled stuttering. It wasn't a relapse in the sense that I
was returning to my old way of stuttering. In fact it wasn't
my old way at all! This was new stuttering and quite different and more severe than the stuttering of my youth. For
instance, I can presently stutter on two or three different
syllables of the same word. I can now stutter while lying
in bed. I can even stutter when talking alone in an empty
room. All of these are new ways that I stutter now that I
never did before.

In the past four years I have often looked back upon
those eight years of fluency. Oh, how I did carry on during
those fluent years! I was as proud as a peacock and had a
brain to match. Stuttering all seemed so easy then. My
fellow tribesmen really didn't need to stutter. There was
a better way of talking and I was the keeper of the keys
that unlocked the secrets of stuttering. But for the past
four years I have been living with failure and defeat . . .
There are now many times when I'm determined to face

my listener and control my spasms, only to find my jaw jerking and my mouth frozen in despair. I had intended to grab the devil by the throat and wring his bloody neck, but instead I'm defeated again. I have sat in the car after one of these episodes and tried to weep, but the tears will not come even though my innards were ready to burst. I hate losing. It gnaws at the fabric of my very being. Losing has, however, taught me the strength and might of my adversary. He is a powerful foe and although I will win some battles I shall never destroy him. I am often bitter that my hard-won fluency was struck down, but perhaps these defeats will teach me of the suffering we all share.

To my more severe stuttering friends who are quiet at the meetings and who don't send letters to *Letting Go*, we feel your pain. We know full well the tempest that boils within you. The hatred, anger and frustration you feel is our common bond. For we too have failed and been defeated, and if you are more severe than us, your pain will be greater and your successes fewer. But know that we are all brothers and sisters and made of the same clay. And we will endure and persevere, for we have fought many battles and although we have suffered many defeats we will not be destroyed.

Carl Dell, Ph.D.
Dept of Communicative Disorders
Eastern Illinois University
Charleston IL 61920

4

Causes

Researchers have tried hard. One might say
desperately . . .

Humans have tidy minds. We like the world to be similarly
tidy. We know that causes have effects, and we like effects
to have causes. We're willing to work very hard, intellectu-
ally as well as physically, to make things fit. We are so determined to find causes for effects that our spiritual and
technological growth down a hundred thousand years has
been fuelled principally by our efforts to discover causes
where apparently none exist. We discovered gravity as a
cause for falling apples. We discovered sin as a cause for
plagues and famines. We discovered germs as a cause for
influenza. We discovered God as a cause for everything.

Stammerers aren't immune to this need. Most stammerers, at some time or another, want to discover the cause
of their affliction. Some say they know it.

One man told me, 'I stammer because my mother was
frightened by a grasshopper.'

Another man said, 'I stammer because I got stuck up a
tree in the garden when I was four years old and for two
hours nobody heard my cries for help. Since then every
speech situation contains for me the expectation of failure.'

Another man: 'I stammer because I talk faster than I
think.'

Another: 'I stammer because I think faster than I talk.'

When I asked a chap I visited up in Wolverhampton why
he stammered, he carefully made no claim to know. But he
did tell me, much later in our conversation and apropos of
nothing at all, that when he'd been in his teens his mother

had said to him, 'I made sure your father didn't do to your young brother what he did to you . . .'

Stuck with an effect as traumatic as a stammer, we understandably arrive at causes by whatever means we can. The man's grasshopper had obviously been a part of his belief system for most of his life, ever since a relative or neighbour told him of it, and had acquired mythic power down the years. The boy up the tree remembered the horror of the event and linked it with the stammer that he probably began to notice at about the same time. His family, similarly tidy-minded, supported him in this.

As to the incompatible relative speeds of thinking and talking, they've been around as long as wheelbarrows, and can be termed 'common-sense' causes. They satisfy by their apparent reasonableness. The man who'd had something 'done to' him by his father was tapping an equally ancient tradition: when all else fails, blame your parents.

I don't want it thought that by offering possible backgrounds to these causes I've intended in any sense to 'explain them away'. Not at all. For all I know they may each be absolutely right. The point I want to make is that they're the *wrong sort* of causes. There are immediate causes, why something happens today rather than yesterday or tomorrow, and there are underlying causes, why something happens at all, and all the above are immediate causes. They're interesting, but they're not what this chapter's about. Nice ordinary people experience them, or nice ordinary people's mothers, and nice ordinary people don't develop stammers. This chapter isn't about stammering's *immediate* causes, it's about its *underlying* causes – the causes nice ordinary people don't have, or they wouldn't be nice ordinary people.

To hammer home the point, a personal experience – one that, as it happens, was also connected with talking quickly.

Some months back, in the course of my research for this book, I was speaking with an excellent local Oxford speech therapist. She was very helpful and friendly, and after we'd discussed her work for a while I was tempted to try for a free personal consultation. I too sometimes wonder about underlying causes, so I turned the conversation to myself, as an elderly, much improved stammerer, and asked her, as the stammer expert, why she thought I stammered even the little bit I did. Not that it bothered me, I said, but it seemed so unnecessary. If I could get so far, whole hours without a single stammer, why couldn't I get the whole way and never stammer at all?

She smiled at me gently, and patted my hand, and suggested that if I still stammered now and then, the reason was simply that I talked much too quickly.

I didn't press it, but I'd been hoping for wise words, profound insights, and it seemed to me at the time a pretty dumb answer. A one-legged man who falls over when he walks quickly, doesn't fall over *because* he walks quickly. Walking quickly is a normal activity. Nice ordinary people do it all the time. It may be the immediate cause of his falling over, but that's only because the poor sod's got something wrong with him. There's an underlying cause. The fact is, he falls over because he's only got one bloody leg.

Similarly (although I admit I'd probably never stammer again if I could only remember not to talk quickly), I still don't stammer *because* I talk quickly. Talking quickly is a normal activity. Nice ordinary people do it all the time. It may be the immediate cause of my falling over, but that's only because I've got something wrong with me. There's an underlying cause . . . Well, it was this underlying cause that I'd wanted the friendly Oxford therapist to tell me about.

Her answer may have been dumb: my question was dumber. Today, with the accrued wisdom of six months' more research, I realise that any half-decent answer would have needed three or four hours, a medical reference library, and a level of basic intelligence from me that my question had shewn her I didn't possess.

In any case, as an experienced speech therapist she'd probably thought she was answering my question's sub-text. No matter what they may seem to be asking, the burning question for most stammerers isn't half so much *why* they do it as how the hell they can stop doing it. So that was the question she'd answered. Don't talk so quickly. And she was absolutely right.

One last word on the subject of immediate causes. They're often quite ridiculously personal. I have a fine example of this from the helpful young man who introduced me to Zarathustra's vision, quoted at the beginning of this book.

He remembers clearly that when, as a little boy, he used to go into his parents' living room at tea time, he'd know at once from the angles of the teacup handles whether he was going to stammer or not, and if he was, how badly. And I don't think you can get much more immediate, or personal, than that.

Obviously, what immediate causes do best is demonstrate stammering's nuttiness. They may occasionally offer clues as to promising treatment approaches, but mostly they're superficial, shop-window stuff. If we're serious about understanding the condition itself, then we must look for what lies beneath them. The python that lives in the house of our speech is only a metaphor. We need a scientific explanation. We need an underlying cause.

As I've already said, there are plenty of contenders for the title.

The first applicant through the door has to be *Stress*. He's plausible and he's a popular contender. We all know that the speech even of non-stammering people, both children and adults, breaks down in stressful situations. We also know that severe and habitual stammering can develop in adults as a direct result of acute trauma – the stress of battle, for example, or of personal disaster. Stress is attractive to therapists as an underlying cause also, I suspect, because its reduction is an easily understood aim, one to which the stammerer readily responds.

Stress has been around as a contender for a long time. Setting aside the calm-down-and-breathe-deeply school of treatment back in the first years of this century, stress was taken seriously among early modern stammering theorists in the 1920s and 1930s – in particular by Wendell Johnson in America. His thinking came to be very influential, and it was based on the belief that stammering in young children was diagnosogenic. He claimed that the disfluencies of children were entirely normal, and would remedy themselves in the natural course of events, as long as attention wasn't drawn to them – in other words, if they weren't associated with stress. If speaking wasn't made into a stressful activity.

In this context a certain Miss Tudor, one of Wendell Johnson's team of young researchers, conducted a revealing and particularly sinister experiment – in Johnson's absence, it must be emphasised. Her work wasn't published at the time, and it's easy to see why.

It wasn't just unethical. It was absolutely monstrous, a scandalous abuse of the researcher's power.

Miss Tudor chose six children, aged 5–15, from an Iowa orphanage, as her subjects. The choice of the orphanage is probably significant: there wouldn't be parents around to ask awkward questions.

All the children were perfectly normal speakers. Nevertheless, at the beginning of the experiment Miss Tudor told each of them:

> 'The [orphanage] staff has come to the conclusion that you have a great deal of trouble with your speech. The types of interruptions which you have are very undesirable. They indicate stuttering. You have many of the symptoms of a child who is beginning to stutter. You must try to stop yourself. Use your will-power . . . Do anything to keep from stuttering . . . You see how X [a child in the institution who stuttered rather badly] stutters, don't you? Well, he started the same way you are starting. So watch your speech every minute and try to do something to improve it.'

On the same day, to the children's teachers and the orphanage staff Miss Tudor gave these instructions:

> 'We have come to the conclusion that these children show definite symptoms of stuttering . . . We have handled a number of cases very similar to these. You should impress upon them the value of good speech . . . Watch their speech all the time very carefully and stop them when they have interruptions. Stop them and have them say it over . . . It's very important to watch for any changes in the child's personality, in his attitudes to his school work, in his attitude towards his playmates . . .'

Miss Tudor visited the orphanage once a month to reinforce these instructions. Unsurprisingly, at the end of four months she was able to describe the children's speech thus:

> All the subjects . . . showed similar types of speech behaviour during the experimental period. All six subjects

were reluctant to speak. Their rate of speaking was decreased. The length of response was shorter. The two youngest subjects responded with one word whenever possible. They appeared shy and embarrassed, and accepted the fact that there was definitely something wrong with their speech. Every subject reacted to his speech interruptions in some manner. Some gasped and covered their mouths with their hands; others laughed with embarrassment . . .

Clearly, in four short months the wretched woman had given the children most of the symptoms of hardened stammerers. We are told that treatment was offered to the children after the experiment (big of her), but that some effects persisted for years.

Dire proof, if such were needed, of the power of stress when applied directly to children's speech: even when, as in this case, the stress is created benevolently. The orphanage staff thought they were helping. They thought they were doing the Right Thing, and there's a fair chance that most of them did it patiently and gently. Yet the final effect was deeply damaging. For once, to paraphrase the old song, it *was* what they did, and it *wasn't* the way they did it.

But it's important, in this chapter on underlying causes, to recognise exactly what Miss Tudor achieved and what she didn't. She gave her young victims most of the symptoms of hardened stammerers. She did *not* give them hardened stammers – at least, there's no evidence in the literature that she did, and I doubt if she'd have been diffident about claiming it if she could have. She robbed them of fluency and ease. Instead she gave them stress, embarrassment, shame. That much was within her power. But their 'speech interruptions', which they'd had all along, she couldn't touch.

So how's *Stress* doing for the job of underlying cause? He comes with good references. On a gut level, too, he makes an attractive contender. He's commonsensical. He's someone everybody's heard of, and he's also perceived by most people to be undesirable. So maybe it's entirely satisfactory that he should be made responsible for stammering, which is also undesirable.

He does have his detractors. There are people who tact-lessly point to the large number of stressed-out children who *don't* stammer; children who are bullied by their parents or repeatedly fall off their bicycles, and yet remain as fluent as a chat-show host. There are people who put forward evi-dence that stress may in fact be beneficial. They tell us its physiological signs are indistinguishable from those of excite-ment, sexual arousal, just having fun. They say that only stress can drive athletes to record-breaking feats. It's stress that makes champions. Furthermore, many actors and musicians only give of their best when half-paralysed by the stresses of stage fright, of ten thousand eager, expectant faces. And not even the most determined stammerer rushes to the window of a burning room, flings it open, and blocks on his cry for '*Help!*' Domestically, too, high stress situations seem to invoke some sort of overdrive: it shames me to remember how fluent I've been during the ghastliest dis-cussions in my life.

All in all, I don't think we can rule out *Stress* at this stage, but I'm not convinced. I don't see him as a natural. One for the short list, maybe.

Next in from the waiting room is *Neurotic Need*, the leader of a whole gang of psyche-based disorders. If we took him on as an underlying cause, stammering wouldn't be thought of any more as inadvertent, just a failure to speak properly. Instead, it would become a purposive activity, something done in order to satisfy an unconscious need. This need might be any one of the many listed in the Freudian alma-nac: aggression, regression, guilt, faeces retention, nipple biting, Oedipal rivalry with the father. It's popular these days to laugh at such notions – they're overused and widely mis-understood – but it isn't easy to disprove them.

Maybe it's their in-groupish 1930s chic that works against them, the Viennese thickness of their jargon. And it has to be said that psychiatrists, in their writings, can be their own worst enemies. For instance, a respected worker in the Per-sonal Construct field, writing sympathetically about the threats a stammerer has to deal with in his everyday life, suddenly comes up with this as her definition of 'threat': 'The awareness of an immediate comprehensive reduction in the number of predictive implications of the personal construct system . . .' I can see more or less what she means, of course, but did she really need quite so many syllables? After all, on the very next page she offers this marvellous revelation: 'Suppose the fundamental thing about life is that it goes on,' she wrote. 'It's not motives that make men do things . . .'

That's one of those thoughts that stays with you, the idea that life might be its own generating force, that things are done for no other reason than simply *because*. It may or may not have very much to do with stammering, but it certainly suggests an author from whom we could all learn a lot – if she'd only let us.

So what about *Neurotic Need*'s qualifications as an underlying cause? Well, our inability to disprove them is nice for him, but it's hardly enough to get him the job. We still have to ask him what he can do for us in terms of understanding our condition, and moving on from that towards some sort of remedy. At least *Stress* points us in what sounds like a promising direction, quitting the rat race, going to live beside a Scottish loch or whatever. Does *Neurotic Need* have anything positive to say for himself?

To be fair, I propose to defer judgment on that point until we've heard from another principal psyche-based contender, *Anticipatory Struggle*. For one thing, he too is hard to disprove.

At first sight *Anticipatory Struggle* seems to borrow much of *Stress*'s equipment, for he claims that stammering is caused by the stammerer's expectations of conflict and failure. He's afraid of stammering, therefore he stammers. At least that's easy to understand. Expecting failure causes stress, and stress causes failure. It's neat. Nicely circular. We know, too, that it works in other fields: the person who walks confidently along a narrow kerbstone will become palsied with anxiety (the expectation of failure) if that same stone is moved to the top of a high wall, and will probably fall off.

But in fact *Anticipatory Struggle* prefers not to rely on anything as unspecific as stress. He likes to invoke 'failure of automaticity' instead. But this too is easy to grasp. Most of our activities – and particularly speech – involve automatic processes. We don't think about what we're doing, we simply do it. Yet even something as basic and bone-learnt as walking can become awkward, even difficult, if circumstances make us aware of it – as when we have to walk across a stage, for example. And the infinitely more complex learnt sequences of music or dancing are more vulnerable still. We're all familiar with the plight of a soloist who suddenly becomes aware of the mechanisms of what he's doing, and so loses it.

It's the guitarist John Williams, I think, who speaks of his fingers having 'learnt' the notes, leaving him to concentrate on the music. They haven't, of course. The learning has been done by those unconscious bits of his brain that work his fingers. But the analogy here is clear. A non-stammerer's speech mechanisms 'learn' the words, leaving him to concentrate on the talking. A stammerer, on the other hand, is constantly aware of his speech mechanisms; he interferes with them, with their automaticity, and his talking goes all to hell. He tenses up, neglects the activity of talking as a whole, and concentrates instead on its parts, its words, its syllables, right down to its initial letters. And in consequence stammers.

Similarly, to take a sporting analogy, the anxious batsman who peers down the wicket, imagining the ball's arrival and rehearsing innumerable tense stabs at it, is likely to put up a catch or get himself clean bowled. And the anxious stammerer, peering at the sentence ahead and imagining the dreaded word's arrival – maybe it's *banana* – is likely to stab tensely at the '*b*' and so miss the word altogether. Words build up into a sentence, just as cricket strokes build up into an innings, and both need to be taken as a whole, and followed smoothly through.

Frankly, I think we've met this applicant for the job of underlying cause before. On that occasion he was called Stammering-is-what-a-man-does-when-he's-trying-not-to-stammer. This time round though, given the proper back-up, he looks a lot more plausible.

Plausibility is all very well. Like *Neurotic Need, Anticipatory Struggle* can make a pretty attractive case for himself. We still have to ask the question, where does his case lead? What positive, on-going elements does it have to offer? And it's here that the prevarications begin.

Since both he and *Neurotic Need* are psyche-based, it's a fair assumption that both would need psyche-based treatment. And the sad fact is that neither psychoanalysis nor any other form of psychotherapy on its own has so far been found to be all that effective. More than that, most reputable surveys have found them to be quite remarkably *in*effective. A detailed study in 1977 of 648 stammerers who had been treated by extended psychotherapy at the New York Speech Institute, for instance, showed that 98 per cent of them had experienced either no improvement or only very slight improvement.

Supporters of this contender might say that this was a comment on the quality of the therapy offered in New York at that time, not on the principle behind the therapy. Unfortunately, similar results show up whenever records are examined closely, and Freud himself – although cautious on the subject (he was cautious on most subjects as he got older) – gives the strong impression that he was finally doubtful about the usefulness of psychoanalytic therapy for stammerers. (For a history of psychoanalytical thinking about stammering, see Bloom L. in the *Psychoanalytic Review*, 1978.)

A further discouragement from giving either *Neurotic Need* or *Anticipatory Struggle* the job can be found in the presumption made by both that stammerers are emotionally disturbed people, and there's absolutely no evidence of this. We've been exhaustively tested for classifiable neuroses of every conceivable sort, and we've shown no deviations from the norm whatsoever.

Researchers have tried hard. One might say desperately. In 1965 – which was perhaps the heyday for the popularity of psychiatric theories for just about everything – a study of primary school children's paintings in the United States indicated that 80 per cent of stammerers had preferred blues and greens to the reds and oranges of the non-stammerers. From this preference the assiduous researcher felt justified in deducing that the stammerers were neurotically reluctant to express their inner feelings. How's that for special pleading? A researcher with something else to prove (me, for instance) could equally well deduce that the stammerers were natural country dwellers, longing for the blues and greens of sky and grass, while the non-stammerers were enthusiastic townies, with a taste for bricks and buses.

No, despite all the researchers' best efforts, they have been unable to come up with a single classifiable neurosis, nor even a single personality trait, that stammerers as a group share uniquely with each other. Not only do stammerers' oddities and eccentricities overlap with those of non-stammerers, but stammerers are often – and this is against all the odds – they are often in much better basic emotional shape. In other words, and I make no apology for spelling it out, stammerers are if anything slightly less nutty than nice ordinary people.

No places on the short list, then, for *Neurotic Need* or *Anticipatory Struggle*. Their case for acceptance rests on the proposition that stammering is in essence the symptom of a personality disorder, and there's simply no scientific evidence to support this. They interview well, but it's all up front: they've had their chance now for fifty years or so and their record doesn't bear examination.

It's time now to look over the candidates who claim that the underlying cause of stammering is entirely physical. Most of them we can send away without even bothering to read their application forms. There's a group of articulatory deficiencies, for example – *Over-long Tongue*, *Intrusive Epiglottis*, *Cramped Lungs* and all their Victorian relatives – that have been exposed as charlatans long ago.

The tongue, in particular, was a favourite guilty party for centuries, plus various surgical abominations intended to make it behave, so much so that the phrase *tangled tongue* is sometimes used as a polite synonym for stammering. It's hard to see how this happened. Viewed objectively, stammering very seldom appears to involve the tongue very much. It sticks out a bit sometimes, but only as a sort of back-up to whatever happens to be the main business. No, if one were looking for an obvious culprit, I'd have thought the lips or the throat were a more natural choice.

Still, we now know that the articulatory bits and pieces of a stammerer are usually in excellent working order, just as good as the similar bits and pieces of non-stammerers.

Another claimant, *Deafness*, is a non-starter. It may result in speech deformities (for obvious reasons), but never in perseverative stammering.

Poor Muscular Co-ordination also doesn't stand a chance. Stammerers' muscular co-ordination, like their articulatory bits, is usually in excellent shape, as good or as bad as that of nice ordinary people. It's talking that bothers them, not threading a needle or playing ping-pong. (In my time I've been pretty good at both these last two.)

There's one applicant, though, who occupies slightly awkward middle ground and can't be dismissed so easily. He's physical, so he belongs in this group, but his workings are mind-based and mysterious. I refer to *Mixed Cerebral Hemisphere Dominance.*

This is a condition that shows up principally in confusions over left- or right-handedness, and it's been around as a possible cause for stammering since the 1920s. It's had its ups and downs – the admirable Van Riper, for one, discounts it – but just at the moment it's enjoying a revival, partly as a result of recent improvements in our ability to measure brain activity in specific regions.

The buzz word here is *dysphemia*, which I began this book with, and which proposes a constitutional predisposition towards stammering, a predisposition that is closely involved with brain function and therefore has entirely physical underlying causes. These causes are hard to pin down just at present – even our improved brain scanning devices aren't yet up to the trillionfold complexities of speech production (maybe they never will be and never should be), but the presence of such causes can be deduced from the symptoms and from what little we do know of the brain's organisation.

We know this much: higher human awareness exists in the big upper fore-brain, which is very much larger than the ancient, reptilian lower brain, tucked away at the base of the skull. This fore-brain is divided laterally into two hemispheres (quarter-spheres really, since the whole upper brain is roughly a hemisphere, but that's not what they're called), and these hemispheres are able to function separately, with responsibility for different tasks. We also know that our principal speech machinery – tongue, jaw, lips, larynx, lungs – are mid-line structures, and that this is less than ideal since it means that they receive their motor nerve impulses (i.e. their instructions) from separate sources in the two cerebral hemispheres – motor nerve impulses that obviously need to be very accurately synchronised indeed if coherent speech is to result. From this fact we deduce that one hemisphere must always be dominant, or conflict may take place. And with conflict will come *a predisposition to speech breakdown*.

(It seems tough, incidentally, that evolution should have come up with this mid-line formulation. Speech is hard enough to acquire without that. How much easier life would be if respiration, phonation and articulation all took place firmly on one side or the other, with no confusions in the chain of command, and a mouth somewhere out by the right or left ear-hole.)

To return to *dysphemia*. We know further that language abilities in both left- and right-handed people are centred in the left hemisphere, while the right, and measurably larger hemisphere is concerned with creativity, with abstractions such as music, and also – perhaps on account of, or as a result of, its greater size – with overall control, also known as dominance. In times of conflict, the ultimate decision-maker. Thus it looks as if the job descriptions of the two hemispheres are fairly clear: the left hemisphere produces language, which the right then converts into speech through its control of the necessary mid-line muscles of respiration, phonation and articulation. This model of the mechanism is supported by studies of stroke victims, where areas of brain damage can be accurately mapped and the symptoms – such as aphasia, loss of language – can be related to them.

As long ago as the 1920s it was observed that a statistically larger percentage of stammerers than might have been expected were left-handed. It was also known by then that the difference in size between left and right hemispheres was less in left-handed people. Obviously the temptation was to connect these two facts and to deduce from them that stammerers were suffering from the efforts of their uppity, unusually big left hemispheres to take control of speech over from their right hemispheres. In other words, so the theory went, the right was exercising inadequate dominance: it was losing control and conflict was developing. No man can serve two masters. Speech can't either. Staff relations deteriorate. Stoppages occur. Unrest. Production breakdown.

Following such a model, therapy in the 1930s and 1940s was often directed towards sorting out this conflict by establishing unambiguous dominance – Victorian ideas of the 'wrongness', the virtual moral turpitude of left-handedness had long been abandoned, so now it didn't matter which hemisphere was in control so long as one was. Results were promising. Left-handed stammerers were encouraged to be left-handed and their stammers improved. Similarly, the fewer right-handed stammerers were encouraged to be left-handed also, on the principle that they were innately left-handed but had been falsely conditioned to right-handedness by their upbringing. The American therapist Dr Eugene Cooper remembers his first job at a school where most of the students he met on his arrival had one or other of their arms in a sling. They weren't, he discovered, a clumsy lot, unusually susceptible to sprains and fractures – on the advice of the chief therapist their dominant hand and arm was being immobilised as part of their having their dextrality changed.

Things got out of hand. *Mixed Hemisphere Dominance* became a catch-all explanation and the cause of every stammerer's problems, to be remedied by the one, catch-all treatment. Unsurprisingly, success rates fell. New theories came along. Dysphemia, as an inherited predisposition, remained a useful idea, but was related to epilepsy instead of to mixed dominance so that for a while stammerers were seen as seizure-prone individuals who were saved from full-scale convulsions by their unusually high blood sugar. This view was supported by statistics that showed many stammering epileptics and few stammering diabetics. Also, the model of a stammering episode as a mini-seizure brought on by stress fitted well with stammerers' own experience.

The years passed. Theories passed also. Therapy results didn't improve and research findings conflicted with each other. In the 1950s and 1960s the psychotherapies flourished, but as we've discovered, to no great effect. Then, in the 1970s and 1980s, *Mixed Hemisphere Dominance* (MHD) staged a come-back, boosted by pre-natal studies which indicated not only that the male sex hormone testosterone retarded neuronal development in the foetal brain, but also that the effect was more pronounced in male rather than female foetuses.

This was music to the ears of the MHD fans, since it explained the preponderance of males over females who stammered and/or were slow to develop speech, as well as the higher incidence among males of language-related disorders such as dyslexia. And it fitted well with even more recent studies, with brain scans that seemed to detect unusual right hemisphere brain activity during stammering episodes, as if unwelcome right hemisphere interference were leading to conflict.

So things today are looking good again for MHD. We must remember, though, that this position has been reached via the concept of dysphemia, which ducks the possibility of anything as specific as a single underlying cause for stammering, and proposes instead a constitutional predisposition. And it has to be admitted that this is an altogether woollier notion.

Perhaps we need a woollier notion. After all, if you link stammering too closely with MHD, and therefore with males of ambiguous dextrality, then you don't have an explanation for those apparently firmly right-handed women who stammer like crazy (there are a few of them), or for those men who don't stammer at all yet are so ambiguously dextrous that they write with one hand, drink their beer with another, and play world class snooker with another. Constitutional predispositions, on the other hand, have room for all these and more. Predispositions guarantee nothing: they're too woolly for that. They provide woolly opportunity and suggest woolly likelihoods.

Looking for safe generalisations, then, it's probably fair to say that many people are born with a predisposition towards stammering, but not all of them go on to develop the full perseverative syndrome. For that to happen some additional influence has to be present. There may well be many of these, but one of them is certainly MHD.

This fits in well with current genetic theory, which similarly limits itself to providing opportunities and suggesting likelihoods. Apart from discrete physical features such as Granny's blue eyes or Uncle Harry's big feet, what we mostly inherit are predispositions. Virtuoso musicians do not invariably, or even very often, have virtuoso children, but they do have children who are very likely to show a predisposition towards music. Stammerers, too, do not invariably have stammering children, but their children do seem to have a predisposition towards stammering that is significantly above the norm.

This view isn't simply anecdotal. Admittedly there are more than enough well-known examples, stammering fathers and stammering sons, stammering Charles Darwin and his stammering uncle, entire inbred stammering villages in the Adirondaks, to create a mythology. But there's more than that. There's strong statistical support for it – in this case the first large-scale systematic pooling of data, made by the North American researcher Andrews and his colleagues back in 1983, that established beyond any reasonable doubt, that the incidence of stammering among first-degree relatives of stammerers is three times higher than in the general population.

(The influence of imitation can be ruled out. It's a popular explanation, but it doesn't work. For one thing, and this is an important point in setting stammering parents' minds at rest, the stammering that young children produce is usually markedly different from that of the adults they might be imitating. Furthermore, by the time they reach parenting age many stammering adults have controlled, or even appear to have lost their stammers. Indeed, a 1978 study in Iowa shows that of 511 children of genetically stammering parents, only 42 had parental models who still actually stammered in the home.)

The genetic model for stammering is supported by the existence of very few documented sets of identical twins, of whom only one stammers. In general terms, if one does they both do. I suppose the sceptics who cried 'Imitation!' just now, will no doubt now cry 'Shared environment!', but they're on shaky ground there too, since there seem to be plenty of non-identical twins, of whom only one stammers – yet these too have undeniably grown up in a shared environment.

The preponderance of men with the affliction provides still further support for stammering as a genetic trait, since genetic theory suggests that men are four times more likely to inherit a characteristic from only one parent, of either sex, than women are.

As an underlying cause, then, *Mixed Cerebral Hemisphere Dominance* has only a partial case to make for himself. He may work *with* a constitutional predisposition towards stammering, but he may also be one of the inherited factors bringing such a predisposition about. For a member of that hitherto long discredited group of broadly physical causes, though, this isn't bad going. It makes him short-list material, I think. Simmering on the back burner, along with *Stress*.

There's yet another candidate who sometimes gets a favourable mention – usually from down-to-earth, no-nonsense, debunking sorts of people. In fact, I've already let his name creep in, coming from their lips: *Environment*.

As an underlying cause *Environment*, no matter how unfriendly, doesn't really have much to recommend him. He's far too vague. You might as well blame the weather. Most people experience pretty rotten environments at one time or another, and most people don't stammer. Even during the crucial speech-acquiring years, from two to six years, there seems to be little correlation between the quality of a child's environment and the quality of his speech.

Even so, I believe *Environment* deserves a hearing – for what he has to tell us about human society, if nothing else.

Environment has a wide reach. Even in this limited, speech-related context he embraces everything from the colour of a Manhattan nursery ceiling to puberty rites in the Amazon rainforest, taking in parents and their assorted successes and failures on the way. So what effects do cultural differences have on speech? The evidence here is copious. It's also conflicting.

An anthropologist, working in New Guinea: 'I have not met a primitive who stammered.'

Another, from the same area: 'I remember hearing of several among the Arapesh.'

One exhaustive study among native American Indians arrived at the conclusion that no Shoshone stammered.

Another, in the same area a few years later, found several; it also found a great deal of embarrassment and distrust before any local villager would admit it.

An expert researcher reported stammering among the Ibo in West Africa as being 'practically a mass phenomenon'.

Another researcher, returning from Borneo and Malaya, reported that there were peoples there who didn't even have a word for 'stammer' in their language.

And so it goes. One traveller hears of dozens of stammering Eskimo, another denies meeting any . . .

The only clear conclusion we can draw from all this is that all over the world the people on the spot are reluctant to talk about stammering, or to be all that truthful when they do. It's a very personal, very traumatic subject, and the information researchers gather about it simply isn't reliable.

Even so, after a generous application of pinches of salt, it still seems undeniable that there are regional differences in the prevalence of the disorder, and that these have a cultural basis. Furthermore, as can be demonstrated, perhaps crudely, by the growing numbers of stammerers in contemporary Japan and North America, the incidence of stammering is a comment on the culture in which it occurs.

In this context I can do no better than quote Dr Bloodstein directly: 'To say that there are many stutterers in a given society is very possibly to say that it is a rather competitive society that tends to impose high standards of achievement on the individual, and to regard status and prestige as unusually desirable goals, that it is sternly intolerant of deviancy, and that, as a by-product of its distinctive set of cultural values, it in all likelihood places a high premium on conformity in speech.'

In the above quote not only does *Environment* get a good showing, but there's also another word that's constantly implicit. Dr Bloodstein happens not to use it, perhaps for fear of being accused of over-simplification by his professional readers, but I have no such qualms. It's a word we're already very familiar with: *Stress*.

All cultural environments induce stress of one kind or another in their members. Highly verbal environments induce high verbal stress. High verbal stress is particularly hard on those with a predisposition towards verbal disorders.

A predisposition towards verbal disorders is arguably genetic in origin and even more arguably connected closely with *Mixed Cerebral Hemisphere Dominance* . . .

Aha. It's been a long and tangled path, but at last it seems that a pattern of underlying cause, or causes, is almost complete.

We've already short-listed *Stress* and *MHD*, with *Constitutional Predisposition towards Disordered Speech* as the concomitant factor. Now all that's needed is a mechanism with good credentials that's capable of harnessing all these in the service of something as variable, as quirkish, as utterly unpredictable as a *Chronic Perseverative Speech Disfluency Syndrome*.

After all, most constitutional predispositions show consistency. Stress doesn't instantly override them. The musical child doesn't suddenly become tone deaf in the presence of the photograph of a policeman. The born athlete doesn't immediately become a couch potato when the teacup handles aren't in the right position. Clearly something very delicate, very unreasonable, very authoritative and atavistic has to be at work if a constitutional predisposition towards disordered speech is to be turned into the notoriously unreliable and ludicrous speech processes of the poor bloody stammerer.

Luckily for the present argument, just such an influence is ready and waiting. It's ancient, it's reputable, and its mechanisms are reasonably well understood. Explaining it takes me back to our earlier discussion of the brain and its evolution.

The large upper fore-brain (cerebral cortex) of *Homo sapiens* is in evolutionary terms a recent development. Beneath its occipital lobes lies the far older and smaller cerebellum, the brain structure responsible for the regulation and co-ordination of complex voluntary movement. This is the structure we have inherited, virtually unchanged, from our irrational reptilian ancestors. As well as voluntary movement, this irrational reptilian brain controls the *in*voluntary. Through our limbic system it controls phenomena such as pulse rate, the adrenalin in our blood, the perspiration on our skin, the dilation of our eye pupils, the griping of our bowels. This irrational reptilian brain is also the seat of our simpler emotions: our anger, our fear, our excitement, our sexual delight, our sense of shared identity within a group, and so our mob hysteria, and it empowers all these with the appropriate physical responses. It's not an inconvenient accident that we shit ourselves when we're really scared. So does the rabbit. So does the lizard. So does the snake. We all lighten ourselves, clear the decks for flight or fight.

So does the snake.

Well, well . . . so does our reptilian ancestor, the snake. Can it be then that the stammerer's spontaneous image of the serpent in the house of his speech is only a coincidence? I don't know. If it is, it's a pretty neat one. For what I *do* know is that it's our tiny cerebellum, the brain structure we've inherited from our irrational ancestors, that is the source of our angers and our fears and our simpler delights, and that it's our tiny cerebellum that is responsible also for the regulation and co-ordination of our speech.

The workings of its circuits are conditioned by heredity, experience, evolution, the Moon in Mars for all I know . . . but the minutest surge in any one of them has profound bodywide effects. Primarily it serves our genetic predispositions, making them manifest. For those of us predisposed to sweaty palms, our palms sweat. For those of us predisposed to acid stomachs, our stomachs pump out acid. And for those of us predisposed to disordered speech, our speech becomes disordered.

It's not surprising that such a recent and delicate skill as speech should be easily upset. Nor is it surprising, given the cultural weight we load it with, that speech should be a particular focus point for the stresses of our social lives. Nor yet is it surprising that the workings of our limbic system, prompted by our ancient and irrational reptilian brain that deals habitually in nuances, the fleeting glimpse of a falling stone that must be dodged, the hint of smoke on the air that brings the nose up and the eyes wide and watchful . . . it's not surprising that this system's reaction to more personal, more sophisticated threats should be directed upon this most personal, most sophisticated of gifts. Even cast-iron non-stammerers have uncomprehended, incomprehensible fears – spiders, or perfectly safe third-floor balconies – that render them less than fluent.

How much more vulnerable, then, is the speech of the man with a predisposition.

We seem to have come up with a threesome for the job of underlying cause that this chapter was aiming to fill. It's clumsy and it's speculative, and no individual member is viable on his own, but each has a sound contribution to make, and together, at least until something better comes along, they seem to fit the job description. Heredity works hand in hand with *Mixed Cerebral Hemisphere Dominance* to produce a *Constitutional Predisposition towards Disordered Speech*, and this predisposition is then activated, via the cerebellum and the limbic system, by *Stress*.

Admittedly the case for accepting this cumbersome team is entirely circumstantial. But stammering too is pretty circumstantial, so maybe they suit each other.

Actually, that's not quite fair. I'm underselling them. You may remember that we sent away most of the other applicants because they'd been around for a good few years and had a poor record as bases for successful therapies. Apply the same criteria to my threefold causation theory and the result is encouraging. Identifiable versions of it, if with differing emphases on the relative importance of its members, have been subscribed to by therapists now for ten years or more. An examination of the resulting treatments will appear in the next chapter. It won't spoil the excitement too much, though, if I leak the fact here that things are looking good.

One final point in this chapter. In my experience – even if they agree with my troika and they very well may not – the best therapists avoid getting hung up on symptoms or underlying causes. Those are for you and me while we try to make sense of a subject that otherwise slips like sand through our fingers. No, the best therapists are primarily healers, and healers are well known to treat the patient first, his symptoms and their causes a long way second.

~

Candles of Joy: *this is a letter from a correspondent in Pakistan, written to the editor of* Letting Go.

Dear Mr John Ahlbach,

Thank you very much for your letters of November 29, 1988 and January 5, 1989, and for all the printed material you sent. I deeply appreciate the detail with which you described for me in your letter how to establish an organization to help people who stutter in Pakistan. Your letter was really encouraging and informative. I am determined to follow the instructions you outlined for me.

First of all, I have given a name to the organization. Secondly, I have put two cloth banners across the road at two different points in the busiest commercial areas of Karachi, stating the purpose of the organization and its gratis services with the address of my post office box.

For the last many days I have been receiving scores of letters from people who stutter with their sad and miserable tales. Some are fed up with their lives due to the daily humiliating experiences they face and embarrassing situations they pass. Some wrote that it is unbelievable that our stuttering can be controlled; they think it is a life-long malady, and it will cease with death only. Some women described their secluded, isolated and painful lives. Some parents expressed their grave worries and anxieties regarding their children's stuttering. I am replying to them with encouraging words, telling them that I was also a severe stutterer, but now, not as much as I used to be. I urge them to endure and to look forward to a brighter future and enclose copies of the material provided by you.

I fully agree with your saying this is not an easy task to start and run an organization, but I am sure that your previous advice will help me to overcome the difficulties.

I want next to create a newsletter like *Letting Go*. I request that you suggest a beautiful name for that newsletter.

Mr John, let me say that still I have not received any encouraging response regarding donations from any Pakistani enterprise. I am meeting all the expenses from my own pocket, and I will keep it on and on until the society realises that stuttering is a speech handicap which creates obstacles in the development of one's social, economic and psychological lives.

Please do not think that I am asking you for any assistance.

The rest of my life is dedicated to serving the distressed and secluded who stutter. I know their pain because I have gone through the same situations and feelings. Life is a short time. True satisfaction and eternal happiness can be achieved by lighting the candles of joy in disappointed and defeated hearts.

K. A. Ghani
Pakistan Stuttering Council
653/14 F B Area, Karachi 38, Pakistan

5
Treatment

. . . comforted by the sight of striped trousers . . .

Natural organisms are staggeringly resilient. We humans are more resilient than most – for one thing, down several thousand years we've had to contend with doctors in addition to all the bugs and germs and hungry jaguars. Good health is clearly our natural condition: our systems defend it tenaciously, and when it's taken from us we fight equally tenaciously to get it back. There's an enormous bias towards recuperation, towards basic survival. It's this enthusiasm for getting better that for so long kept doctors looking good – this, and the irrational part of our natures that likes long words and is comforted by the sight of striped trousers.

Certainly, if doctors had to rely for their livelihoods solely on the effectiveness of their treatments, they'd have died young even more frequently than their patients. Not one in ten of their remedies, so it now seems, can have been in any direct physiological sense beneficial.

Take bleeding. There can't have been very many patients whose health was improved by the loss of blood (most will have been weakened by it), yet for centuries doctors' reputations were sustained by their use of bleeding as a cure-all. Obviously enough of their patients recovered despite the treatment for them to get rich and famous.

Maybe it was their bedside manner that did the trick, the black bag and the furrowed brow, backed up by the medical degree, the framed certificate (often spurious) on the wall. Maybe these worked hand in hand with the patient's natural resilience, and wish to believe, to produce results. Obviously something did, for doctors prescribed and patients got better often enough for a connection to be drawn between the two events – an unsound connection, but one sufficiently convincing to justify money changing hands in large quantities.

Sadly the history of stammering treatments is less simple. Adult stammering is one of those ailments – melancholy is another – that goes against the general rule. Although grotesquely counter-productive, once it has arisen it hangs on, or is hung on to, with remarkable determination. It becomes, as it were, the patient's natural condition, from which any departure seems to be vigorously resisted. We now believe, in fact, that chronic stammering can be ameliorated only by awesome endeavours, simultaneously on several fronts, from both patient and therapist.

So how did the stammer doctors of the past stay in business? Partly, I suppose, they were helped by the spontaneous remissions. Many of the more punitive treatments will have worked against these, but presumably a few did still occur. Tenacious though the word-snake is, when he decides to go, he goes. More than anything else though, early therapists, particularly those in the 'stammering schools', must have survived not on their results but on the sheer desperation of their clients – on the belief that any expense, any treatment, any humiliation, no matter how ludicrous or apparently ineffective, was preferable to the abandonment of hope, to the bleak acceptance of their dire condition. As Van Riper puts it, remembering his youth, 'When one stutters terribly and there is no other recourse in the world, one will put up with any folly and endure anything for the hint of hope.'

So the stammering schools sold hope, dressed up with whatever happened to be the particular gimmick – swinging Indian clubs, maybe, or vegetarianism – which they backed up by implanting the truly evil notion that any failure to speak fluently would be entirely the patient's fault, the result of idleness, inattention, deceitfulness or masturbation. This was a technique that lingered. Even as late as 1971 one British teacher was writing of his method: 'The only likelihood of failure lies in a half-hearted attitude on the part of the stammerer.'

I have no words to express the anger this kind of comment can make stammerers feel. First, because it's manifestly untrue. No one therapy will ever be right for all stammerers, and even the right one for a particular stammerer will be far from infallible. Second, because stammerers live with failure: it's a constant corrosive, a deathly part of the air they breathe. Anything that increases it needlessly, unjustly, is a crime.

As well as selling hope boosted by fear, the stammering schools must also have prospered on stammering's notorious tendency to go into temporary remission. The most excessive performer has his 'good' days, even his 'good' weeks. Records of follow-ups are rare. And it would have taken a brave stammerer indeed, as an ex-student, to protest publicly should he suffer a relapse, hung about as this would have been with admissions of failure and immorality.

The most excessive performer, too, can achieve at least a fleeting fluency if he adopts a novel manner of speaking. The Victorians knew this, so they practised 'Rhythmic Stimulation' of one kind or another, an imposed regularity of speech that was achieved by syllabising and pausing, and the systematic clustering of phrases. As late as the 1960s you could buy a behind-the-ear metronome, the Pacemaster, and the principle is still practised today. Another hoary favourite, 'Regulated Breathing', produces much the same effect. Both can produce stammer-free speech, but only for as long as they're employed – and the speech they produce is so odd that few people care to persevere with it for long. I've already quoted Van Riper's 'cured' fellow-student, whose speech sounded like that of the living dead.

Equally temporary was the improvement reported by one researcher in America when his subjects spoke while crawling round on their hands and knees. In fact, to cut a long story short, I can probably do no better than to go back to Dr Bloodstein: 'Somewhere, at some time, almost any therapy can achieve a remarkable result for some stutterer.'

For how long, however, is another matter. Another North American therapist, Dr Eugene Cooper, warns his patients: 'There are no quick fixes.' And relapse is never to be taken lightly. It's more than simply a return to the former condition: all too often it's deeply demoralising, yet another perceived failure, yet another nail in the coffin of the stammerer's hopes, his self-respect, his dignity.

I'm afraid none of this seems to have advanced the present discussion very far. A definition of a stammer has been suggested, and a team of probable causes, and we've established what may realistically be expected from a cure. Now we must look at the principal possible treatments presently available and try to understand what they have to offer – not to Dr Bloodstein's 'some stammerer, some place, some time', but to your average, run-of-the-mill stammerer (if such a creature exists), any place, any time.

The field is large, and I cannot emphasise too strongly the fact that, since no two stammers are the same, no one therapy can be expected to have the same effect on them. At the most basic level, any therapy that significantly improves the patient's sense of well-being, his confidence or his peace of mind, will reduce the severity of his stammer. All too often, though, these are transitory responses, and they're unreliable indicators when considering a particular therapy's lasting usefulness for a particular patient. For some patients the simple fact of being in therapy, of having a sympathetic ear to bend, is enormously beneficial. Others, for whom the therapist represents change and therefore threat, will need to persevere before they see any improvement.

The catalogue that follows isn't intended as a sort of home shopping aid, from which the stammerer may choose the therapy that suits him. Choosing therapies is a professional's job – home shopping, even for such basics as shirts, is a perilous business: all too often the contents of the parcel that arrives are a nasty disappointment. No, the purpose of this list is simply to make the stammerer aware of the main current therapeutic approaches, some of their advances and some of their pitfalls, and perhaps to help him, when he has sought out a professional, to know roughly what to expect and to answer her questions wisely and well.

Most of this information is directed principally at adult stammerers. Parents of disfluent children who are seeking advice might helpfully read it for background material, and then turn to Chapter 6, which is specifically devoted to them. There are organisations, listed in Appendix 2, that will advise them further. Every expert recommends prompt action if a child's speech gives any cause for concern: in ninety-nine cases out of a hundred the disfluencies will be normal, a natural stage in the child's development, but in the hundredth case, when a potential stammer is diagnosed, an early response is the best way to maximise the chances of nipping that stammer in the bud.

POSSIBLE TREATMENTS

Self-help

The most popular option among adult stammerers is probably to go it alone, with the aid of some book or manual, tape or video. These may well be misused or misunderstood, and actively damaging (such material is almost invariably intended to be no more than a companion to expert hands-on therapy), but they offer the great advantage, being a private transaction between them and the stammerer, of sparing him embarrassment or humiliation. The stammerer doesn't have to expose his infirmity to the cold light of another's scrutiny, and if there are unpleasant truths he doesn't want to face, he doesn't have to face them. Also, self-help is cheaper than visiting a private professional therapist – but if it doesn't work, and it usually doesn't, then it isn't cheap at all, and a waste of time too.

My belief is that little can be said on behalf of the going-it-alone approach. Its only clear advantage is that it gratifies the stammerer with the warm feeling that he's doing something about his affliction – what more could anyone ask? – while in fact requiring him to do absolutely nothing. But in this context Stevenson's travelling hopefully isn't enough: most people don't know that he went on to point out, 'The true success is to labour.'

Success rates in this area are obviously very hard to guess at. Nevertheless, the significant lack of endorsements for it from AFS members, coupled with professional therapists' views on the subject, suggests that very few stammerers have been significantly helped simply by reading a book, listening to a tape, or watching a video. Even if exercises are proposed and undertaken, the necessary stringency is usually lacking – the will may be strong but the flesh in such matters is notoriously weak. It needs encouragement, it needs support, sometimes it frankly needs bullying, none of which a book or tape or video can provide.

Furthermore, no one mail order or bookshop treatment can possibly suit all stammers. Undertaking a 'cure' without expert advice is as risky as any other form of unskilled self-medication. The stammerer may be lucky, but the chances are he'll waste his money – and his time, if he takes the treatment's instructions seriously. In which case his stammer may well end up worse than it was to begin with, since he's had another failure to add to all the rest. This is something he can well do without – too much of the stammerer's life is already filled with totting up failures, and the degree of his fluency is closely bound up with the state of his morale.

Hypnotherapy
Hypnotic suggestion, which has been used to treat stammering since the beginning of the nineteenth century, is another attractive therapy. First, because it's undemanding: a cheque is written, after which all further responsibility is shifted firmly from the patient to the therapist. Secondly, because it's known to be effective in other, possibly connected fields: for one, in the curing of cigarette addiction, which some doctors believe may be quite as much a matter of perseverative behaviour allied to image-building as it is of a physical craving for nicotine. And thirdly, because nobody quite understands how it works – which makes it an ideal treatment for a condition whose workings nobody quite understands either.

(People who discuss hypnotic states, and how they're induced, sometimes use grand phrases like 'subcortical filtering', but in reality careful electroencephalograph studies of subjects in hypnotic trances show their cortical brain waves to be indistinguishable from those of their waking state. All that can really be said is that some sort of partial cortical inhibition must take place, such as that which enables a mother to remain totally alert to the crying of her child, while apparently sleeping soundly.)

The attractions of hypnotism as a treatment for stammering are largely delusory. Its record isn't good. For one thing, by no means all people are capable of being hypnotised. For another, although those stammerers who are so capable often find their speech much improved, the benefits are usually very short-lived. A clinical investigation of hypnotic suggestion with forty stammerers was reported in the *Journal of Speech Disorders* in 1946. Of the forty, nine didn't respond adequately to hypnosis. Twelve spoke fluently while in a trance but didn't respond to post-hypnotic suggestion. The remaining nineteen spoke fluently both during and after the trance period, and reported that their speech continued to be fluent for two or three days following hypnotic sessions – but for no longer. This study refers to a group of stammerers each of whom was worked with repeatedly for a period of at least seven weeks.

Stammering isn't like cigarette addiction. It isn't a conditioned reflex either, which, if overcome for a week or two, will genuinely cease to exist. Stammering is a bone-deep impulsion, the product of infinitely complex mental and physiological forces. The most powerful of these forces, in the adult stammerer, is almost certainly his long-established anxiety about his speech which a hypnotist's brief reconditioning can do little to overcome. Confidence may be instilled at the time of the session, and even carried forward in the susceptible for a while by means of post-hypnotic suggestion, but it's entirely superficial. Nothing important has changed. Beneath it the same old life-long needs and insecurities grumble on. Only the slightest countersuggestion of failure is needed before they all come scrabbling through.

At any rate, this is what the record suggests. Dramatic improvements have been seen. Even in the unpromising conditions of hypnotists' stage shows, such as those of the famous Emile Coué, severe stammerers have been induced to address the audience at length, with total fluency. Stammerers have been similarly transformed by eating goat turds or getting punched on the nose. Nobody says how long the transformations last, though, and the probabilities aren't encouraging. Those follow-ups that have taken place suggest that no significant success rate can be attributed to hypnotism on its own as a treatment for stammering. Coué, for one, reports a stammerer he 'cured' who appeared at a speech clinic within a week, stammering more severely than before.

Which is not to say that there are no able, well-trained and responsible medical hypnotists around. Of course there are: they do important work in many fields, and their help can very usefully be enlisted as part of an overall treatment. But be wary of the small ads: to quote an experienced and delightful Canadian stammerer, among the ranks of the professional 'hypnotists' there are 'enough quacks to stock a duck farm'.

Suggestion

None of the above should be allowed to discredit hypnotism's older brother – not as a sole cure, perhaps, but certainly as an important factor. The power of suggestion has always been central to most forms of contributory healing, and today that fact is widely accepted. Even a technical skill such as dentistry is more easily employed if the patient feels at ease in the chair and can believe that his dentist loves him. How much more potent then, in coping with the less definable ills that beset us, is the expertise and optimism radiated by the successful medical doctor in his surgery, or the speech therapist in her clinic? The profession calls this the 'therapist factor', and it's as personal as fingerprints, as indefinable as a sense of humour.

Inevitably, not every 'therapist factor' suits every patient. I can remember one therapist driving me mad with the way she hitched her skirt up just half an inch – never enough to make any real difference – before she crossed her legs. Nevertheless, she was an excellent therapist, very successful with people who didn't mind the little hitch between each crossing of the legs. This is why no stammerer need fear that he's going to cause hurt feelings if he decides that he and his therapist just aren't hitting it off. She's wiser than that, and she's been there before. He should worry, though, if he's on his third or fourth therapist and they still aren't hitting it off. Maybe he's not yet ready to hit it off with *any* therapist.

Returning to the therapist factor, I'm reminded, in a slightly different context, of my early married years and of the book on childbirth my wife and I both read. At that time the most popular childbirth guru was a Dr Grantley Dick-Read. His book was calm, informative, encouraging. Only in one aspect did it give us cause for doubt: Dr Dick-

Read stated categorically that in his experience there was no pain in childbirth. No pain, only mild discomfort.

Was he lying? Certainly his opinion seemed at odds with all the available first-hand, if anecdotal evidence. Was he a charlatan? Surely not: his reputation was good and on every other matter his views seemed sound and sober. His picture on the book jacket was of an unusually gentle, wise and honest elderly gent. No exaggerator, no purveyor of false, sales-building promises . . . We decided the crucial phrase in his statement was 'in my experience'. In his experience, with him at the bedside, with his hand on the clammy brow, with all that gentleness and wisdom and honesty, we could well believe there'd be no pain. It wouldn't dare. He wouldn't allow it, only mild discomfort. Evidence, we'd say now, of a powerful therapist factor.

The pains of a course of stammering therapy are slightly less than those of childbirth, but they're to be reckoned with and they last longer. To get through them the patient needs to be given faith: faith in his therapist and faith in himself. He'll probably have neither to begin with; he'll need to be given them. Enter the therapist factor. He may know, objectively, that his therapist is excellent, with a long, successful record; he may also know, objectively, that he himself is an excellent fellow, very worthy of her attention. But knowing isn't believing. It isn't faith. It won't sustain him through his coming labours, the tiny gains, the huge discouragements, the eventual reshaping, with any luck, of his entire identity. Only faith will do that – the faith his therapist gives him that he and she together are capable of such things.

Not that faith alone will lastingly move the mountain of his stammer. But without faith, if I may dare another biblical paraphrase, all his therapist's exhortations will be as sounding brass or a tinkling cymbal.

Relaxation

An excellent stress reducer. Never harmful, usually beneficial. And I'm taking relaxation here to include all similar consciously achieved states. The tranquil centring of yoga, for example, the physical harmony aimed for when practising the Alexander technique. The measured otherness of Zen Buddhism. All these disciplines, and many others, shape human efforts in one way or another towards a sense of personal well-being. More specifically, they are concerned with something I can best call peace, and so they would seem to me particularly appropriate to the treatment for something I can best call war. For that's what stammering is, a state of permanent conflict between intention and execution, between the speaker and the serpent in the house of his speech.

Put simply, it's just not possible to remain relaxed and to stammer, in any usual sense, at the same time.

Relaxation's sense of personal well-being lingers. It sets people up, sometimes for the day, sometimes for even longer. Similarly, whether it's induced by music therapy, breath training, therapeutic dance, meditation, a good therapist, or post-coital torpor, there's a carry-on effect that results in stammerers being able to speak more fluently for a while afterwards. But the length of that 'while' is unreliable (where have we heard this before?), and is also extremely variable between subjects. Some manage to stay as it were semi-relaxed for long periods, to the benefit of their fluency. For the rest, life's little difficulties quickly jangle and the relaxed state falters, particularly at those loathsome moments when we would most prefer it not to.

Relaxation helps the stammerer. It helps him as much, and no more, than it helps everybody else who's willing to practise it conscientiously. As a specific for his stammer, however, on its own it's unlikely to do much.

Pills
With the development of tranquillising drugs in the 1950s, the clear connection between stress/anxiety and stammering gave many therapists the hope that such drugs would provide the ideal treatment. Banish the stress/anxiety with tranquillisers and the stammer goes too. Perfect. The logical solution. Unfortunately, as with many other apparently logical approaches to stammer therapy, the results have been disappointing.

There *are* stammerers who have been lastingly helped by tranquillisers, but most simply sit around, stoned happily out of their minds, stammering fit to bust. Banish the stress/anxiety with tranquillisers, remove the censors, the shame and the embarrassment, and more often than not the stammer blossoms.

Possibly what this most suggests is that we're mistaken when we bracket stress and anxiety so automatically together. As I've already shown, under certain circumstances stress works wonders for the stammerer. It's fair to say that anxiety never does. Anxiety is the real, all-weather killer. And if that's the case, then surely anti-depressants, the drugs most often prescribed for anxiety states, are the answer?

Yes indeed . . . except that these tend to have hyping-up side-effects that stammerers can absolutely do without. As so often happens for the poor old stammerer, it looks like a no-win situation.

Various sophisticated drugs have been tried – haloperidol, propranolol, meprobamate, oxprenolol, for instance – and various drug cocktails. Each one of these sought a different approach. Propranolol has been found effective against essential tremor. Oxprenolol improves skilled performance under stress. Haloperidol is thought to block dopamine receptors in the nervous system. All these, and many others, have produced real if limited improvements in some stammerers. Little as these are, though, they don't persist after the drug therapy is discontinued, and very few patients have thought it worth continuing at the cost of their becoming habitual drug users. As one-off zappers, just to get someone through a particular job interview or whatever, they may have value, but their use is very risky. Haloperidol, for example, can cause noticeable drowsiness, a quality not likely to impress a prospective employer.

The mention of cocktails leads me smoothly to the most obvious drug of them all, alcohol. Once again, there's no clinical evidence that stammerers are less disfluent when drunk. Their disfluencies probably worry them less, which is nice, but that's the most that can be said. Even their cheerfulness is notoriously short-lived, and furthermore comes with unhelpful after-effects.

Vitamins have been used in stammering therapies, particularly B and C, often in large injected doses. If they make the patient feel better, which they may well do, then well and good, but it's very hard to imagine that they can have any direct effect upon his stammer. The same goes for the whole gamut of alternative medicines. Interestingly, in the 1960s Soviet speech therapists used a treatment very close to acupuncture and reported good results . . . If such approaches help, and sometimes they undoubtedly do, then in the absence of firm clinical evidence (most alternative medicines are still not being taken seriously by research scientists), I believe that the improvement in the patient is probably general rather than specific. And while this is obviously an excellent state of affairs, it seems to be as unpredictable for the stammerer and as liable to relapse as any of the others.

New drugs and compounds will certainly be devised and tested. Personally I think it's unlikely that any disorder as clearly multi-causal as stammering will respond to them.

Finally, in May 1992, according to an *Independent* news report, American scientists were injecting stammerers' vocal cords with botulinum toxin – a substance responsible for severe, even lethal food poisoning, that kills by paralysing lung and heart muscles – and by this means were successfully reducing the stammer. It sounds drastic. Presumably they weren't reducing their patients also.

British specialists are considering trying out this treatment – but only in very severe cases where adults have developed stammers as the result of brain injuries or strokes. Dr Lees, consultant neurologist at the National Hospital for Neurology in London, says he already treats a rare condition known as spasmodic dysphonia (strained, strangled speech) with the botulinum toxin, injected three or four times a year through the Adam's apple under local anaesthetic, and admits that the treatment 'is not pleasant'. Maybe that's why only the worst stammering cases will be asked to put up with it. Certainly, as a stammer therapy, it's still very much in the experimental stage.

Actually, the piece in *The Independent* is not seriously to be trusted. Not only does it spell vocal 'chords' somewhat bizarrely throughout, but it also points out that the toxin anyway 'does not get to the root of the problem in those with speech defects which are thought to result from a chemical disturbance in the brain'. *A chemical disturbance in the brain*? If that's so, then it's the first I, or any of the people I've talked to, have heard of it.

Psychotherapy
In its narrow sense the treatment of neurosis according to formal psychiatric theory, i.e. psychotherapy, has a poor record of success with stammerers. This isn't surprising: Chapter 4 on Causes establishes that stammering is generally accepted not to be a neurotic condition, and that, according to all the tests, stammerers are an impressively non-neurotic group of people. Not that they never have neuroses – such a group doesn't exist – but the neuroses they have just aren't directly connected with their stammers. Thus conventional psychotherapy on its own is not applicable.

As Dr Bloodstein tells us, 'The absence of conclusive research evidence that stuttering is an attempt to satisfy unconscious needs, or that it is wholly or necessarily a symptom of personality conflict, does not make for confidence that future efforts to treat it through psychotherapy will be more successful [than today's].'

Broaden the sense, however, to include the popular term counselling, and psychotherapy's back in business. After all, counselling encompasses help in everything from how to deal with your incestuous impulses to how to face up to your low stature or your loneliness. So why not your stammer? Counselling is what we all do when we respond to someone's appeal for advice, but professional counsellors are trained, with their intuition ideally left intact, to do it better. Counselling, at its best, is a grown-up, face-to-face, dogma-free transaction, and that ought to place it at the centre of any approach to healing, whatever the disorder.

This is not to say, however, that counselling on its own is likely to be of more than passing comfort to your actual hardened adult stammerer.

Already in this survey of stammering treatments, when doubting the effectiveness of this or that one, I must have used the phrase 'on its own' four or five times. Inevitably therefore, the discerning reader – and aren't all readers discerning? – will be ahead of me, galloping on to the obvious conclusion. I'm afraid I must ask him or her to be patient. No doubt I'll get there eventually – a multi-causal affliction will presumably be found in the end to require a multi-pronged therapy – but in the meantime there are a few more specific treatment approaches that deserve to be seriously considered.

Behaviour Therapy

There is a wide range of behaviour therapies. None of them, unlike psychotherapy, is much concerned with underlying causes. Accepting the non-neurotic theory of stammering, behavioural therapists attack the affliction entirely through its symptoms. They see maladaptive behaviour and they attempt to modify it. How they go about this depends on how they think the maladaptions occurred in the first place.

Some behavioural therapists believe stammering to be basically a fear response. All sorts of irrational fears plague all sorts of people. Stammerers come at a very early age to fear speech. They wish to speak but they also wish to avoid speaking. The psychospeak for this dilemma is 'approach/ avoidance conflict', and there's plenty of evidence that it plays its part in the stammerer's bag of tricks.

First he sees a difficult word or situation coming up ('difficult' in the sense that it's given him trouble before, which makes this a ridiculously circular process), so he focuses an unnatural amount of tension in his speech organs. Already, therefore, he's making life difficult for himself.

Second, he focuses on the first letter or syllable of the word, again because it's given him trouble before. This further stacks the odds against him – non-stammerers think in whole words, not in their separate components.

Third, he starts doing all this (to the extent of preforming the sound in his mind and even with his lips) well in advance of the predicted difficulty, thus making it virtually certain to occur.

This idiotic sequence of events was first observed and analysed by Van Riper. He called it the 'Preparatory Set' that a stammerer constructs for himself, and he constructed his own therapy very much with the aim of breaking it down – that and a technique of crafty negotiation with the stammer snake, rather than blunt confrontation, that I'll be getting to later. I've seen two very long video tapes of his treatment sessions with a young stammerer (they're intended for student therapists and they're available on loan from the

AFS library service) and they're very impressive – if only for the powerful 'therapist factor' the old man radiates.

Further support for fear as a motivating force in stammering – or anxiety, if fear is thought too strong a word – can be found in the research done into the hierarchy of stress figures who measurably influence a stammerer's difficulties. This can be listed, in diminishing order, across a very large number of patients as: 1) the boss, 2) strangers, 3) parents, 4) grandparents, 5) casual friends, 6) close friends, 7) spouse, 8) siblings, 9) children, 10) pets. This is such a reasonable pecking order, and so much what one might have expected, that it gives a definite boost to the approach/avoidance conflict theory.

Therapists following this line take the fear to be phobic, a classically conditioned response, and try to modify it through classical desensitisation techniques. As with the phobic fear of spiders, that we're told can be eliminated by repeated, carefully monitored exposure to the beastly things, so the phobic fear of speech is to be eliminated by the repeated presentation, often fantasised, of stressful speech situations within the reassuring, low-anxiety atmosphere of the clinic or consulting room.

This is inevitably a lengthy process. The research findings show that, when practised on its own, it helps most stammerers a little but very few stammerers a lot.

Instead of fear as the motivating force in stammering, other researchers have seen the affliction simply as a learned response. The problem here is that for a response to be reinforced (i.e. learned), it has to be seen in some way as advantageous and it's hard to imagine what advantages stammering can ever have been seen to bring in its train. I'm not at all convinced by the suggestion that a child gains enough attention from his stammering to make him want to persist with it, nor that it's useful to him as an excuse for other inadequacies or failures. More devious is the suggestion that stammering gets reinforced by the decrease in the stammerer's distress once his block or gargle is over. That sounds to me like a rehash of the old story of the loony who bangs his head against the wall because it's so nice when he stops . . .

Next in the line of behavioural therapies is 'operant

conditioning'. This is a polite way of describing therapies which bash the stammerer, in one way or another, every time he stammers, and I have to admit that they have more than the statistically predictable number of successes. Patients who receive electric shocks, blasts of sound through earphones, verbal abuse, punches on the nose, or even financial penalties, do seem to stammer less – at least for the period of the treatment. (Van Riper reports a man who claimed his stammer was cured when he was a child via regular applications of his father's leather belt to his backside.) How on earth such stress-inducing conditions could possibly help something that's supposed to be a stress-induced disorder I haven't the faintest idea, but if that's the cure you want, then go for it!

Another form of operant conditioning, by rewarding moments of fluency rather than punishing moments of disfluency, is sometimes used with children. Large quantities of ice cream or candy change hands, or tokens with which toys can be bought, and a fat greedy child results, but sadly there's very little evidence that they do much for his stammer.

Yet another way to modify stammering as a maladaptive speech behaviour is to follow the Victorians and impose upon it artificial restraints of some kind. Building on the well-known short-term effectiveness of assumed funny voices, foreign accents, unnatural rhythms and the like, several hi-tech approaches along those lines have been tried.

Anything that slows a stammerer's speech is likely to be helpful. Behind-the-ear metronomes do this. So do traditional syllabification and artificial breathing techniques – and also modern masking effects such as the Edinburgh Masker. This last, an anonymous sound ('white noise'), is transmitted through headphones to the stammerer sufficiently loudly to prevent him hearing his own voice. As a result of this he tends to speak more slowly, to shout a bit, and to stammer much less. Most stammerers don't get on with the Masker, but a few have been helped considerably. In the 1970s a refinement of this effect was developed. Called Delayed Action Feedback (DAF), in it the headphones receive the subject's voice from an exterior microphone and play it back to him after a short delay – anything from 50 to 300 milliseconds. Used under clinical conditions, DAF produces (sometimes after a period of confusion in the patient) a marked improvement in his fluency. Whether this is in fact because of the delay, or because of his slower speech rate, or simply because all the gadgetry distracts the patient from his stammer, nobody seems to know for certain. But DAF is a part of many therapy programmes these days, and gradual reductions in the length of the delay are used to habituate patients to their newly fluent speech so that considerable carry-over can be achieved. DAF is also unique among the behaviour modifiers in that the speech it produces sounds fairly normal – most of the others result in such peculiar, I-am-a-Dalek type speech that you'd have to be a pretty desperate stammerer before you'd resort to one of them.

Should you have a spare £595 + VAT (the 1991 price) available, there's a neat little personalised DAF device on the market that offers a tickly bonus – it returns your speech to you not only through headphones but also via a vibrotact-ile transducer strapped round your neck. The literature rec-ommends that the headphones are for use 'only in the clinical setting or in the privacy of your home or office'. The 'vibrotactile feedback', however, is unobtrusive in ordinary day-to-day use and will help you to 'slow your speech' and avoid 'locking your vocal cords' (whatever that may mean).

The manufacturers are disarmingly honest. 'The equip-ment does not provide a magic cure,' they warn. 'However, with your commitment and with professional guidance, combined with a training programme, you can achieve more control over your speech production.' It's a modest claim. The fact that it can be successfully marketed, at such a price, with such modest claims, is a humbling comment on just how desperate many stammerers may be.

Latest among the behaviour modifiers is electromyo-graphic (EMG) feedback. This is one of the many loosely-termed biofeedback techniques by which subjects learn to bring under their conscious control bodily functions that are usually unconscious – blood pressure or pulse rate, for example. When applied to stammering, EMG feedback enables the patient to monitor his own muscle tension in the speech-producing areas of larynx, chin and upper lip. When the level of tension is reproduced via surface electrodes as an audible tone, the stammerer quickly learns to reduce it.

Until mid-1992 properly documented clinical tests had been limited to very few patients, so optimism must be muted. Nevertheless, five sessions of learning and practice had resulted in patients being able to maintain low muscle tensions and stammer-free speech, with no further use of the gadgetry. And the effect still persisted nine months later, when a follow-up was undertaken.

These are early days. EMG feedback technology is elaborate and expensive. New approaches that seem to work are always over-exciting. It would be nice though, and not entirely implausible, to imagine a day, maybe in seven or eight years' time, when the technique is standard and is helping hundreds of thousands of stammerers.

Finally, from one of the latest stammering-as-behaviour modifiers to one of the earliest. Back in the 1920s the thought occurred to several therapists that they should not so much be trying to defeat the stammerer's snake as negotiating with it. Instead of treatments directed towards 'curing' the stammer, which brought with them assumptions that stammering was a bad thing and that frankly any degree of disfluency was socially a disaster, the new approach aimed at convincing the patient that stammering wasn't really so bad but that maybe there were better ways of doing it.

There's sense in this. Certainly in most social situations the listener's distress is a response to what he sees as the stammerer's distress. It's not the stammer that embarrasses nice ordinary people half as much as the stammerer's embarrassment. Once you succeed in breaking that circle, in which the stammerer's emotion produces the listener's emotion, which then feeds back to intensify the stammerer's emotion, then his disfluencies often become much less severe.

There are strong elements of psychotherapy in this approach (making the patient feel good about his stammer and therefore about himself), but it's also robustly concerned with the practical mechanics of the thing. Once the patient can concentrate upon trying to stammer fluently, which is possible, rather than upon not stammering at all, which is usually impossible, then a great weight of failure is lifted from his mind. He can begin to find out exactly what he does, and look for less obnoxious ways of doing it.

For example, a stammerer formerly disposed to astonish his listeners with six loud 'amah's before he got round to amah-amah-amah-a-mother, may find that some discreet humming, mmmmm-mother, will satisfy his stammer snake just as well. Or at least the therapist can suggest this to him and see how he feels about it. There's no commandment that says, Thou shalt not negotiate.

The gains are enormous. The stammerer's disfluency will be genuinely less obnoxious, so he will feel less bad about it. Therefore his listener will feel less bad about it, so the stammerer will get back good vibes, at which point his anxiety levels will be reduced and he may even find himself able to invoke his mother with no accretions at all.

For a decade or so, in the 1950s and 1960s, this approach went out of fashion. It was seen as an admission of defeat – which in a limited sense it was and still is – and the experts forged ahead with all guns blazing, aiming to blast the snake right out of his lair. But the fact is, as many of them have now realised, if you've shot off all the shells you've got and the enemy's still eating well and sleeping well, it's pretty stupid not to admit it. Indeed, it's mostly through admitting defeat that you can start to go forward again.

This doesn't mean that therapists should simply give up, and settle for teaching their patients to live with their speech difficulties as presented. It also doesn't mean that, even with our admittedly limited present knowledge, recovery is impossible. It particularly doesn't mean that schemes working towards all-out victory shouldn't constantly be pursued. It just means that until some sure-fire winning therapy comes along there's no harm in boosting the chances of the present ones with a little negotiation. With learning to stammer fluently.

And even then, as Van Riper emphasises, nothing's easy. A total push is needed. An attack from every quarter, with every weapon. He suggests one hour's individual therapy, plus one hour's group therapy, three days a week, plus regular practice in between, for anything up to four months. Other therapists will set different targets. None will deny that a major effort is needed.

Self-help Groups

In the stammering community – a variegated gang notorious for its communication difficulties – it's not surprising that self-help groups have a hard time. Making arrangements for get-togethers isn't easy when most members would choose to stay at home rather than face using the telephone. Committee meetings tend to be thinly attended, and even then they tend to drag on a bit if people insist on having their say. Groups get started, falter and fade away.

Even so, on the local level some stammerers' self-help groups do survive surprisingly well, and on the national level they prosper. Maybe one stammerer in a hundred is a group-minded person, and luckily that's just enough. Nationally – as with the British Association For Stammerers or the American National Stuttering Project – groups concern themselves with wide issues, with educating public attitudes and resisting misrepresentation, and they're often militant. Locally, the concerns are naturally more parochial, with district health facilities, for example, and also, most importantly, with individual problems and individual needs.

Simply going along can be a revelation. For many people a problem shared is a problem halved – to know that you're not alone, that other people are just as weird as you, or weirder, and to be able to talk about (stammer about) your difficulties openly without shame or embarrassment, and to know that they'll be understood in an unsentimental way that only fellow-sufferers are capable of, is a great morale booster. Some groups are led by speech therapists, who give their time and energy and skill with unstinting generosity. Others are entirely lay. Some groups may consist of no more than three or four people who have met often enough to become friends. Others are plugged into the national network and run regional events, cricket matches, charity walks, stammering workshops. All do valuable work, and all run the risk of becoming ghettos, warm and snug – non-judgmental environments in which people who have previously hidden from society can continue to hide, people who will travel round from group to group and workshop to workshop, professional stammerers who choose the sheltering comforts of the group above the more demanding rewards of the world outside.

I don't think this matters. Puritanical exhortations to self-improvement, to facing up to reality (which in this context is always for some reason unpleasant), are easily made. Beyond a certain point, I avoid them. We deal with our infirmities as best we can. If a stammerer is helped by going to a professional, good luck to him. He may be losing out somewhere else, but I haven't heard of any holy stammer-serpent law that says he shouldn't do what he can. We all lose out on something or other.

As to self-help groups as a therapy, however, I believe their effect can only be extremely marginal. Maybe they help self-confidence a bit. Certainly they provide an information service – and a way to spend an evening now and then that leaves you feeling you've done something constructive and even slightly virtuous. And what's nicer, for heaven's sake, than feeling slightly virtuous? But as an actual remedy for your actual stammer, self-help groups are a wash-out. Join one, and work your fingers to the bone for it. I hope you will, but if you want serious help with your stammer, go and get some proper therapy. And by 'proper' I mean therapy from a professional, properly trained therapist.

Therapists

I have a very high opinion of speech therapists. Those working with adult stammerers have a particularly hard row to hoe – the adult of the species often makes demands upon them far beyond the call of duty – but the entire field of treating speech and language disorders is extraordinarily exacting. Patients suffering from neurological damage following head injuries, for example, may present serious disabilities that are all the more distressing because they are basically incurable: the thrust of any therapy has to be towards helping the patient to adjust, devising strategies for coping, giving him or her back some sort of confidence in the possibility of communication. It's a task that requires caring of the very highest order.

In Britain, the speech therapists' professional governing body is the College of Speech and Language Therapists. There were schools for deaf mutes before the end of the eighteenth century and – as I've already shown – in Victorian times treatments of one kind or another were devised for a wide range of speech and language disorders. But it was a ram-shackle, quack-ridden business. Perhaps the one thing in all the world that the obscene trench warfare of the First World War can be thanked for is the change it brought about in attitudes, both public and official, towards speech disflu-encies. No longer were these seen as comic, or reprehensible, and for the first time the need was recognised for specialist skills in treating the relentless parade of fighting men, whose skulls had been torn open or their nerves shot to hell, on their return from the front. Their desperate plight moved even the Whitehall authorities, and 'speech correctionists', otherwise known as 'instructors in vocal therapy', were called in to help.

Although these came from markedly different back-grounds – some were teachers of singing or elocution, some had been trained to teach the deaf, others had worked in hospitals coming along behind the neurologists, plastic sur-geons and ear, nose and throat specialists – they all shared an interest in speech disfluencies and a willingness to learn from each other. Many men were helped by their work: many, through the gift of hope, had their lives literally given back to them.

The important discovery made during those years was that, with proper treatment, these men *could* in fact be helped. In the matter of 'proper treatment', however, the plain fact was that most of the therapists were working by guesswork, and that some sort of professional training was urgently required. Shortly after the war, training schools were established: connected to major London hospitals, they offered two-year courses for 'remedial speech trainees'. And in the 1920s London's Central School of Speech and Drama set up a separate speech therapy department, providing a full three-year course. The hospital approach was different at this time from the drama school approach, more clinical and less emotionally intense: nevertheless, speech therapy as a medical discipline had officially arrived, and with it the title 'speech therapist'.

In 1929 the first School of Speech Therapy was opened at the West End Hospital in London, and others quickly fol-lowed in Liverpool and Glasgow. This growth of the speech therapist's respectability may in part have derived from public knowledge of the stammer of the Duke of York, soon to be King George VI. After his sufferings in his closing speech at the Empire Exhibition in Wembley Stadium in 1925, relayed by radio to a global audience of some ten million people, the Duke had received treatment from an Australian speech therapist, Lionel Logue. Logue's notes of his first meeting with the Duke have often been quoted:

> He entered my consulting room at three in the afternoon, a slim, quiet man with tired eyes and all the outward symptoms of the man upon whom habitual speech defect had begun to set the sign. When he left at five o'clock, you could see there was hope once more in his heart.

Later, Logue said of the Duke, 'He was the pluckiest and most determined patient I ever had.'

Not that Logue ever 'cured' the Duke's impediment – my own recollections of the King's radio broadcasts in the 1940s are of struggles I recognised only too well – but as a result of his very public and courageously faced difficulties at least it was never again possible in Britain to write off all stammerers as battle-scarred wrecks or incompetent nincompoops.

The Second World War also brought its own crop of head injuries and shell shock. The army employed trained speech therapists, and by D-Day in 1944 there were seven of them on active service. Not many for so great a fighting force, perhaps, but a great advance on the previous war's none.

The year 1944 was also the time when the therapists' various professional associations recognised their shared aims and (mostly) shared techniques, and amalgamated to form a single organising, controlling and examining body – the College of Speech Therapists.

Useful official recognition came in 1945, when children with speech defects were among those handicapped children for whom local education authorities were required to provide special education treatment. A year later the National Health Service Act of 1946 recommended the general employment of speech therapists in hospitals. Since then, speech therapists have built themselves a professional structure separate from, and independent of, the medical profession – a discipline in its own right, responsible for its own clinical decisions, career organisation, training and regis- tration. Their success has been reflected recently in the creation of three university professorships in speech and language therapy, at City University, London, the University of Newcastle-upon-Tyne, and Queen Margaret College, Edinburgh. And in April 1991, the governing body of the College of Speech Therapists recognised the increasing amount of work its members were doing in the field of lin- guistics, and changed its name to include Language in its title. Not as small a change as it seems, for it recognises the enormous progress made during the last decade in under- standing language structure and the complex mechanisms that convert thought into word.

As well as providing a regulatory body for its members, the College lists many other aims in its literature. I think they're worth detailing here, if only to hearten my fellow stammerers with the large amount of work being done on their behalf. The College has recently moved to a grand new building, where it plans to establish a resource centre that will include the following facilities: information systems with on-line access to relevant databases; reference books and professional/academic journals; samples of current assess- ment and treatment materials; facilities for viewing pro- motional and demonstration videotapes; rooms fully equipped with audio-visual facilities for holding meetings for clinical and research speech and language therapists, thera- pists in education, managers, and client groups.

The College is also committed to the development of clini- cal practice through research − in particular it believes that adequate methods of evaluation need to be developed which will accurately reflect the aims and objectives of speech and language therapists, and the needs of their clients. Addition- ally, the College publishes an impressive list of books, manuals, and leaflets, not all of which are addressed to its expert members: two leaflets, in particular, are invaluable for the parents of young children: *Are you worried about your child's speech?* and *Does your child stammer?* There's also a very useful Directory, listing the names and addresses of current members of the College, and the addresses of clinics through- out the country, together with the therapists working at them. And finally, if you can plough through it, the College's reprint of the Education Act 1981 for speech and language therapists is a revelation. The parents of a stammering child have legal rights they probably never dreamed of. I don't say they'll get them, but there's no harm in trying.

On the subject of research, and separate from the College, the Association for Research into Stammering in Childhood has recently been set up as a registered charity. As its name suggests, it aims to specialise in stammering's beginnings, the crucial early years when we now know most disfluencies can be remedied if they're wisely handled. Its organisers believe that in Britain children who stammer, and their parents, are seriously neglected and that they urgently need professional guidance. Provision for specialist help for pre-school and school-age children is very limited indeed, and what little help there is will be jeopardised by the reorganisation of the Health Service.

Accordingly the ARSC plans to provide assistance for stammering children, and ultimately to establish a centre for intensive treatment and support for children who stammer and their families. As is being recognised increasingly in the United States – the Southwest Texas State University is particularly active in this regard – the treatment of stammering in children is a family matter and needs to be taken whenever possible into the home.

In the short term, the ARSC hopes to reduce waiting lists for children needing assessment and treatment – the 9+ months common at present in Britain makes a mockery of the need for early treatment – and they aim to involve the family of the stammering child, thus continuing the work of the speech therapist in the home environment.

In the long term, the association's aim is to educate and inform teachers, youth leaders and others working with children, of the special problems stammering brings, and to fund and promote research into the means by which stammering may be prevented and treated, and to disseminate the results of such research for the benefit of the public.

For stammerers there couldn't be more valuable work. As the ARSC points out in its literature, 'A stammerer who has not been successfully treated in childhood usually has a serious problem for life.'

*

So the College of Speech and Language Therapists directs and regulates the profession. What, then, can you expect of the therapists it represents? The first thing to understand is the wide range of communication difficulties they are qualified to treat. Working closely with other medical and psychological professionals, they provide help not only to stammerers but also to patients with learning difficulties, all degrees of impaired hearing, aphasia caused by strokes or head injuries, to patients recovering from plastic surgery, and to patients with voice or articulation disorders. They assess children's slow speech learning and other language problems, and help the elderly with a large number of communication-related handicaps.

Typically, a therapist will spread herself round many jobs: she may on different days of the week attend a hospital or health centre clinic, a school language unit, a child assessment centre, a geriatric home, a rehabilitation unit, as well as supervising evening group sessions and treating patients on an individual basis, perhaps in her own home.

Her qualification for all this is a three- or four-year undergraduate course, often followed by two years of postgraduate studies. Sixteen polytechnics, colleges and universities in Britain currently offer accredited courses, and this number is steadily growing. All courses are comprised of theoretical and clinical elements. It's an impressive list: *Psychology* – normal and abnormal developmental processes and behaviour, and psycholinguistics. *Phonetics and linguistics* – analysis of speech, voice and language and their mechanisms. *Anatomy and physiology* – neuroanatomy and the specialised organs serving oral communication and hearing. *Language pathology and therapeutics* – description, assessment, diagnosis and treatment of communication disorders.

Other elements include acoustics, audiology, disorders of ear, nose and throat, education, neurology, orthodontics, plastic surgery, research methodology, statistics, and sociology . . . On top of which there are skills in patient care to be acquired, inventiveness in devising varied activities for patients young and old, and of course, finally, the vital, but unlearnable 'therapist factor'.

So the therapist you meet in school or consulting room or clinic has formidable skills behind her. Also, she's doing something she believes in passionately – she's overworked and underpaid and she wouldn't be there unless she did believe in it. She'll put a considerable investment into your case or your child's, and she'll expect a similar investment from you. It's the only way, frankly, that anything'll get done.

The College describes her work like this: 'Speech therapists work with children and adults who have communication difficulties for a variety of reasons – physical, mental, social and emotional. After assessing the nature of the problem, speech therapists use their theoretical and practical skills to rehabilitate, educate and counsel patients and their families, with the aim of reaching as great a measure of independent communication as possible.'

It would be presumptuous of me to try to put it better.

~

A letter to the journal of the AFS.

As parents of a stammering child we have endured many sad and funny incidents with his speech. Our son's stammer became apparent when he was three years old. The doctor said, 'Leave it alone and it will go away'. We did, but it didn't go.

When embarking on his school career (age five) the teachers were completely thrown – could he read or not? They had obviously not come across a severe stammer before. With a large class there was no time to find out so he was sent for remedial help reading lessons. I was horrified, as I knew he could read and understand words far beyond the level of most 5–6 year olds . . . Finally the remedial teacher gave him a practical test and discovered that his vocabulary was excellent and he shouldn't be wasting her time in a remedial class.

Now he is off to secondary school this September and I know he wonders how he will keep ridicule at bay. I have advised him that he won't. First year pupils at a new school are always a target but I have tried to explain that if boys want to be offensive they will, and the boy who is too tall, too small, too fat, or has extra thick glasses will be upset just as much as a stammerer.

As to what the future holds, who knows? We are told there is no miracle cure but it has to come from within. Maybe as he gets older he will be more aware of how important all the little tips from the speech unit are, especially after attending an Intensive Stammerers' Course in London for two weeks in the Easter holidays which provided lots of helpful hints and practical help. It was also quite an experience to meet other stammering children and their parents and share their hopes and aspirations.

6
Parents and children

*We've come a long way from the white-coated dragon with a
pocket full of pens . . .*

Though life is hard on the adult who stammers, I believe it is
even harder on the stammering child – and therefore maybe
hardest of all on his parents. Often, in the early years, before
he goes to school and the pressure on him begins, the child
will hardly be aware that he's disfluent. There are many
more interesting things for him to think about. But his
parents will be aware. And because they love him and want
the best for him, they will worry.

It is easy for parents to over-react if they have a young
child who shows signs of disfluency. They cannot bear the
thought that he may be handicapped, less than perfect in
some way. After all, on a deep level all parents want their
child to be perfect and successful because he is an extension
of themselves: his failure and imperfections are in this sense
their failures and imperfections. In fact, if parents were
honest they would probably have to admit that they hope
their child will turn out better than they did, and so make
up for their own inadequacies.

Most parents sensibly manage not to let all these needs and
anxieties show – growing up is tough enough for children
without that – but the feelings will still exist, and they are
powerful. They are necessary, too, in moderation: without
them no child-rearing species on the face of the earth would
survive. If protective mechanisms get out of hand, though,
they may do more harm than good.

For a child's parents his speech is of particular significance:
it is his interface with them and the world, his expression
of self, his means of becoming a person, and it is very easy

for them to let his smallest disfluency trigger an excessive reaction. They will often deny their distress, hide it and pretend that everything is fine. They may also panic, and metaphorically run screaming into the street. But neither response is helpful. They are right to be concerned, but only in so far as it prompts them to seek expert advice.

The statistics are reassuring. Over half the children in the industrialised world (where research has been undertaken) show signs of disfluency at one time or another during the early years of their acquiring speech. It's absolutely normal: a stage a child naturally passes through. It's also normal that a few of these children will develop clinically identifiable stammers. The vast majority of these stammers will go away, without treatment and permanently, over the next few years. Only a very few children – one per cent of the entire population – develop stammers that persist and require therapy. And of these few, therapy will cure many and help most.

In short, it's very unlikely indeed that any young child's hesitant speech, repetitions, stumbles or mispronunciations are signs of a lasting stammer. They are much more probably a normal part of the process of learning, of discovery and differentiation, that all children go through.

This is most definitely not to say that they should be completely ignored. They are matters for reasonable concern. Given any doubt at all about their child's speech, parents should immediately seek professional advice. No matter how long the odds are against the need for therapy, where a child's future stammer-free speech is concerned they're not worth gambling on. There's everything to be gained and nothing to be lost.

The Association For Stammerers issues well-prepared leaflets of basic advice; so does the College of Speech and Language Therapists. Their information is clearly presented, with a sensible lack of technical language. They explain the child's possible problems and they recommend ways in which parents or carers can help. And the first recommendation is early referral. In the words here of the College of Speech and Language Therapists: 'Parents should contact a speech therapist as soon as they are concerned about their child's stammering. Don't waste time. Don't be diffident.

Don't be afraid that people will think you're making an unnecessary fuss. They won't. Somewhere near you there's a doctor, a health visitor, a teacher, a play group leader, someone who'll be happy to put you in touch with a trained speech therapist. It's your right under the law.'

The Association For Stammerers emphasises the part played by the parent: 'Wherever possible a speech and language therapist should be contacted so that parents may be supported and the development of stammering prevented.'

Notice the priority: at this stage it's the parents who have the problem – the child is almost certainly blundering happily on, quite oblivious. Furthermore, if anything needs to be prevented it's *'the development of stammering'*, not the disfluencies he's presenting, which may well be quite normal.

It's important, also, that speech therapists shouldn't be imagined as formidable or frightening, either to children or parents. We've come a long way from the white-coated dragon with pince-nez, clipboard, and a pocket full of coloured pens – if she ever existed. Wherever the first assessment takes place – in your home, in play school, at a clinic – your child will have little idea of what's happening. The therapist will want to see him completely at his ease. She's interested in the whole child, not just in his speech. She'll talk to him, but there'll be no open concern with the way he answers, certainly no 'putting it into his head' that he may have a stammer.

The therapist is highly trained: in particular, her skills help her to spot the subtle differences between a child's normal disfluencies and a stammer. If, after the assessment period, she has her doubts (in most cases she won't have any) and thinks that the child may after all be on the way to developing a stammer, the treatment she will offer is more likely to take the form of advice to his parents rather than direct treatment for the child.

A few decades ago it was quite common for parents to be blamed for their children's stammers. This is no longer the case. The experts may not know much for certain, but they do know that parents on their own absolutely cannot make a child into a stammerer.

That is not to say that some parents won't go out of their way to invent guilt for themselves. The mother of a friend of mine is a typical case: she steadfastly believes that she caused her older son's stammer by never letting him suck his thumb. It's a claim she makes whenever the subject comes up. She also believes that when she let his younger brother's thumb-sucking go uncorrected she caused his sticking-out front teeth instead. This is a true story. Some people seem to need guilt. Maybe it's just that they need life to be parcelled up into neat little packages of cause and effect, guilt and innocence.

The fact is, on their own parents cannot make their child into a stammerer. On the other hand, they can undoubtedly help him not to become one. And that's where the trained therapist comes in. She's able to suggest many well-proven ways of helping the young potential stammerer.

The advice she will give is likely to be in the areas of increasing the child's confidence and reducing communicative stress. If you talk quickly yourself, for example, your child may feel he's expected to do the same and so end up stammering because he can't quite manage it. In that case, a simple reduction in your own rate of speech may well be all that's needed.

In any event, the speech therapist is the person you need. Parents on their own have a good record in helping children with their disfluencies – witness the many stammers that go into permanent remission without expert treatment – but unfortunately there are always a few children for whom their parents' love and common sense aren't enough. And it's these children whom the speech therapist has spent four years in a college learning how to help.

Remember also that the speech therapist will always err on the safe side. As a result there may be children she helps whose disfluencies would have gone away anyway, without her intervention. But nobody can ever know that for sure, and certainly her advice can't have done any damage, so there's everything to gain from consulting a speech therapist.

Despite everyone's best efforts, there will be some children whose stammers persist. Nobody knows exactly why this is. We only know that there are stammerers who will stammer no matter what. No therapy offers guarantees, and no therapist either. But the chances of success, or at least of great improvement, are excellent – especially if the disfluency is treated early, before stresses develop around it, before habits form, and a stammering pattern becomes established.

Unfortunately those very few children who do become long-term stammerers cannot be recognised in advance, despite the considerable research that has been carried out into the early causes and origins of stammering.

Way back when I was growing up, before the Second World War, the comforting word went round that stammerers, as a group, were of above average intelligence. This wasn't just sucking up to the parents – researchers had produced statistical evidence. Didn't someone once say that there were lies, damn lies, and statistics? Still, in this case they seemed quite sound – they'd been drawn from a study of quite a large group of young people, and they showed that the stammerers possessed significantly higher IQs than the non-stammerers.

Unfortunately for the theory, however, the study turned out to have been conducted within the competitive, closed society of university students, so of course the stammerers were brighter. All that proved was something that stammerers had known all along: to succeed in any competitive environment – and perhaps particularly so under the harrowingly verbal demands of university entrance – it was necessary to be brighter than the norm. Women have the same problem. In a man's world their basic nature works against them. In a fluent world stammerers' basic nature works against them too.

So, as a group stammerers simply aren't significantly more intelligent than nice ordinary people. Nor are they significantly dumber. Admittedly there are other studies (aren't there *always* other studies?) that turn up a larger than expected number of stammerers among the mentally deficient. But many of these subjects are reported to be unaware of their disfluencies, which introduces another factor: since they had no impulse in childhood to deal with such disfluencies, nobody can say exactly how relevant these people are to the overall picture. All in all, the general conclusion appears to be that stammerers are well represented at both extremes of the IQ spectrum, and at all points in between.

Other attempts to separate out stammerers have been

equally unsuccessful. Apparently a stammerer isn't an only child more often than the norm, or more subject to allergies, or fatter, or thinner, or more neurotic, or less neurotic, or more subject to encephalitis, or slower to acquire bladder control in infancy, or more likely to have suffered abnormal birth conditions. This odd-looking list is in fact a random selection from the countless aspects of our physiology and psychology that have been studied in vain for signs of commonality. Researchers are a determined and ingenious lot. In manual skills, in general bodily co-ordination, in motor capacities of the speech musculatures, in visual acuity, in auditory thresholds, in biochemical factors, in psychosexual fixations, in suggestibility . . . in all these areas they've found that stammerers pan out just like everybody else.

In 1932 one study came up with an amazing observation that nobody so far has been able to (bothered to?) disprove. The test results demonstrate beyond all reasonable doubt that stammerers – wait for it – that stammerers make many more errors than non-stammerers when they're asked to respond to recorded announcements of three-digit numbers by writing them down with the first two digits reversed. I'll say that again, in case you missed it. No I won't . . . The fact is, researchers are indeed a determined and ingenious lot. And indeed, considering recent research into the significance of MHD, possibly in this case they may actually have been on to something.

One thing they do tend to neglect though, for all their ingenuity and determination: they seem to take no account of their test subjects' motivation. I'm reminded of a research project that was undertaken in order to measure the relative aspiration levels (that's ambitiousness, not breathing) of male and female stammerers. Using a research device called a Rotter Board, which is a sort of modified pin-ball machine, the researchers arrived at the conclusion that male stammerers had higher levels of aspiration than female stammerers. They don't appear to have considered for a moment the possibility that men might simply be more willing than women to play damfool pin-ball. Similarly, might not non-stammerers for some reason be more willing than stammerers to spend their days writing down three-digit numbers with the first two damfool digits reversed?

One final example of the things researchers get up to on the stammerer's behalf. It concerns Oral Stereognosis, which is the name experts give to a person's ability to recognise solid shapes that are placed within the mouth. A 1981 study established beyond all reasonable doubt that stammerers were less good at it than non-stammerers. A nice ordinary person's mouth is apparently cleverer than mine at telling safety pins from paper-clips, or whatever.

I shouldn't knock it. Stand up that boy who said all knowledge had to have an application. And in any case, nobody knows what wondrous application may not be just around the corner.

Of course all this mass of research is well-intentioned and in a good cause, and of course it would be a marvellous breakthrough if stammerers could be found different from non-stammerers in any basic way other than in their rotten speech. For one thing, it would provide a focus for treatment, the starting point for a theory, and a general area in which to begin looking for a treatment. It would also enable stammerers to be identified earlier in their lives, and so get them treated better, sooner.

Until this happens, therefore, all manner of research should be supported, no matter how bizarre, and today's catch-all, better-safe-than-sorry approach should meanwhile be followed: it mostly works, provided that parents are watchful, and willing to ask for help.

So what then are the sorts of disfluency parents may find in their children, and how may they be expected to develop in the child with a clinically diagnosed stammer?

I shall rely here on a unique investigation conducted and reported upon by a leading American authority, Dr Oliver Bloodstein, who followed the progress of 418 stammering children in great detail from the ages of two to sixteen. His report breaks the development of their stammers down into four phases, at the same time emphasising that although these may be typical they're definitely not invariable. Any child may skip one, regress, or even compress all four into a year or so.

Phase One The pre-school period, between the ages of two and five. The most significant quality of the stammer within this phase will be its episodic nature. It appears for fairly brief periods – a few weeks or so – between long periods of fluent speech. It may be quite severe, and will consist principally of repetitions of short words or phrases, usually at the beginnings of word groups, and it occurs most often when the child is excited or upset. Although he is often aware of his difficulty and may even be frustrated by it, the child basically isn't all that concerned. He's interested more in what he wants to say than in how he's saying it. Getting held up in what he wants to say is what bothers him: not anything deeper.

It's during this phase that the majority of spontaneous remissions occur – the fluent periods lengthen and the stammering episodes eventually don't return – and it's during this first phase that the therapist's advice is most likely to produce results.

Phase Two This is a four- or five-year period during which the condition becomes essentially chronic. There are no longer any fluent periods. The child is aware of himself as a stammerer, but is still fairly unconcerned. There are few attempts to avoid difficult words or situations. The stammer is worse under conditions of stress, and typically occurs throughout sentences rather than simply on initial words. Remissions are rare now and the therapist's work is much more difficult.

Phase Three By the time the child is ten or eleven years old his stammer will have become integrated into his life. He will think about it. He will understand that it is more trouble in some situations than in others, and may take avoiding action. The actual stammer itself may take any form – blocks will have arrived by now, and irrelevant body movements – but he still regards it more as an inconvenience than as an assault on his identity or a cause for shame. At this stage changes in family attitudes, a sensible reshaping of family reactions to the child's difficulty, may still be enormously helpful.

Phase Four This phase is characterised by its obsessiveness. In his adolescence now and on into adulthood, the person is in many respects ruled by his stammer, and a full range of substitutions, avoidances and irrelevant movements is in play. His stammer is a serious problem to him, and he's likely to be hypersensitive to the reactions of others. He often regards his stammer as shameful, refuses to discuss it, and goes to great lengths to appear a normal speaker. As a teenager he will suffer from all the inevitable pains of adolescence, plus stammer-induced guilts, uncertainty, and fear.

As Dr Bloodstein himself emphasises, the above is a dangerously neat account. It must not be taken to mean that progression from phase to phase is regular, predictable, or inevitable. It can accelerate. It can also stop – or be stopped – altogether.

Neither should this measured, efficient-sounding description be taken to mean that anybody understands the mechanism behind it. Nobody does. There are guesses, apparently good ones, and I'll be going into them later. But nobody knows for certain exactly what happens, why or how.

We know quite a lot about what stammering isn't; very little about what it is. Although serious scientific research into the subject has been going on now for upwards of a century, many experts in the field would say it's still woefully inadequate. One leading American speech therapist, Dr Eugene Cooper (we've already met him in Alabama), operates a clearing-house for international stammering research. He reports a very meagre flow of material, maybe three or four items a month, and for what little information there is, no central data bank exists.

In an excellent 1984 book the Australian researcher Dr Roger Ingrham wrote:

> There is an almost desperate need for a data base from field clinicians on current stammering therapy procedures. If clinicians could be encouraged to gather and report data ... the profession would be considerably advanced. For only clinicians can show the strengths and weaknesses of treatments in the field, rather than in the research laboratory.

In passing, I have to admit here that it seems to me that what little information there is sometimes gets framed for purposes of obfuscation rather than illumination. How about this, from a couple of respected Minnesota researchers who report that stuttering appears to be associated with 'temporary recurrent reduction in the dynastic control of the super-adjacent levels of the central nervous system over their substructures, causing general disequilibrium of the orientation potentials with the nervous system necessary for efficient speech'. I suppose that's how professionals talk to each other within most disciplines, but I wish they wouldn't.

In any case, you mustn't be afraid that your local speech therapist will hit you with stuff like that. I'm guessing of course, but I suspect that the most she'll want to tell you is that present knowledge suggests three kinds of factors that make up a child's disfluency. There are predisposing factors (heredity), precipitating factors (upsets, illnesses, losses), and perpetuating factors (insecurity, stress, unsuitable demands). Little can be done about the first two – we all get a mixed bag of inheritance and we're all bashed around a bit by life now and then – but the third group, the perpetuating factors, are a very promising and hopeful area. Therapists and parents (and siblings too) can get together and genuinely make some progress, co-operating in the disorder's early stages and so lessening the chances that stammering will become established. The prognosis is good. Families really can help.

Meanwhile, more research is taking place. In Europe and North America visionary stammering projects are under way. In Britain the Association for Research into Stammering in Childhood (ARSC), has recently been established, as a charitable foundation with the specific aim of setting up a centre for research and treatment. Its committee is advised by leading speech therapists and child psychologists, and includes stammerers and the parents of stammering children. All these people, through personal experience, have recognised the need for such a centre. ARSC is fund-raising actively at the moment, and has produced a short video film, *Time to Talk*, introduced by the actor Michael Palin, which movingly demonstrates young stammerers' problems and suggests ways in which they can be lessened. By contacting this association plus the other organisations listed in Appendix 2 of this book, parents will find a wealth of information that will help them to deal positively with their child's disfluency.

~

The following advice is taken from an AFS leaflet addressed to the parents of a child who stammers. It's as sensible and down-to-earth as everything else the AFS does, and I believe that anybody who may ever have to talk to a child, whether a stammerer or not, can learn from it – and that surely means *everybody*.

What can we do to make speaking easier for a child?

> *Look at the child and get your face on the same physical level.

> *Speak in language that can be understood easily.

> *Talk about the present and about things that can be seen.

> *Reduce the number of questions that you ask, allow the child to choose when to tell you things.

> *Give the child time, slow your own speech, show that you're interested and listening.

> *If the child is very disfluent, then reduce demands. Maybe return to some of the favourite books, rhymes, games and activities to help the child feel the security of the familiar.

7

Conclusion

. . . what's left sounds awfully electrical . . .

I've tried to avoid making this book autobiographical, the story of my stammering life. But now that I've arrived at my final chapter, and at the need to look ahead and even maybe make some positive contribution, I find that unfortunately my personal experiences will have to creep in. For it seems to me that, while the entire weight of stammering research is, and has always been, concentrated upon the patient's moments of disfluency, my own experience suggests that a study rather of the patient's moments of *fluency* might be surprisingly fruitful. No matter how rare they may be, all stammerers *do* have these moments, and in my case they used to come with a very curious and distinctive sensation. Other stammerers I have talked to seem to recognise this sensation, so it must be reasonably common, yet I've never found it written about or heard of it being studied.

I think it should be. To prepare the background, therefore, a synopsis of my stammer's early days:

Family folklore has it that by the age of four I was stammering briskly. Nobody, of course, knows why. My parents had separated and departed when I was a tiny baby, but whatever trauma this may have caused was ameliorated by a very loving (and wealthy) grandmother who welcomed me into her rather lonely life – she was widowed – and brought me up tenderly . . . with the assistance even of a real-life nanny, in real-life sensible nanny's shoes, who was fond also, and stayed around in fact until after I'd left school and gone away to National Service. I go into this simply to emphasise that, although I was fatherless, I cannot believe I was all that emotionally deprived. My mother, who was an actress, visited quite often. She was an awe-inspiring figure certainly, but doesn't – indeed, shouldn't – every young life have one?

In any case, the important aspect of those early years, as with many young children, is that my stammer didn't bother me. I have not the slightest recollection of it – other than a memory of my mother, on one of her visits, telling me, 'If I stammered as much as you I wouldn't talk so much!' But that's neither here nor there. I was a chatty, cheerful child, and I remember no troubles at all when I went off to my rather posh little kindergarten, even though I've always understood that my speech was very disfluent at the time. No doubt privilege buys these advantages – my class was tiny and the teaching 'enlightened'.

At eight and nine years old I still don't remember stammering. I remember grown-ups gently suggesting that perhaps I should take a deep breath and start again, but I remember no actual moment of stammering, and certainly no distress.

At about this time I went off to my first speech therapist. He was a kindly old gentleman in a dark striped suit with a waistcoat, and he got me to read aloud to him – great long lines of fusty verse, Matthew Arnold it may have been – which I could always do perfectly fluently anyway. I don't know how long I went to him, not very long I suspect, but he taught me breathing exercises on his shiny black leather couch, which I played at afterwards in bed, but they never seemed to have anything to do with my stammer, and he also gave me the one useful anti-stammering tip I ever heard. He suggested that if I got stuck on a plosive 'b-b-b-', putting an 'mmm' in front of it would get my mouth into the right shape and lead me into the 'b' nicely. It worked, and I've used it ever since.

By the age of ten, and at a prep school, my stammer had become a bore. I could still read aloud fluently though, even in class, and teachers were tactful about asking me questions, and I don't believe the other boys teased me. Still, it was a bore getting stuck on things, usually the most important words, and I do remember trying to stop my head from jerking around. But I was a bit of a buffoon, and an unquenchable performer: if I stammered I could always horse it up a bit and get a laugh, and maybe that was my way of coping. And at twelve I entered a reading aloud competition and won a prize. I was unstoppable.

I think I was already getting the curious sensation that this story is about, but I can't be sure.

Outside the sheltered school environment, of course, life was very troublesome. Bus conductors, librarians, shop assistants, telephones, these posed all the usual threats and mostly I avoided them. I never asked the way (I still don't), I didn't go into cafés, I got someone else to buy my model aeroplane kits for me, I didn't talk to any strangers I didn't absolutely have to.

School was fine. There was another stammerer there, a red-faced boy called Bamford, with very blond eyebrows – whatever happened to Bamford, I wonder – and the general attitude to our problem was friendly. Foreign languages presented the worst difficulty. Attempting actually to *speak* French or German (my best subjects) reduced me to a twitching wreck (it still does). But my written work was OK and I was a passable Rugger second row forward, and you can't have everything.

And besides, my performing was going places: not only could I read aloud with fluent and histrionic fervour, I'd discovered that I could also act in school plays. As long as the words were read or learnt, not my own – ad-libbing was totally out – I could talk just like everybody else. I got decent parts in end-of-term plays and I read lessons in the school chapel. I was Somebody. More than that, to people who didn't know me I was just another nice ordinary person. Because of course, under all the razzmatazz, I hated, hated, *hated* being a stammerer.

Meanwhile, therapists came and went. None of them helped me, and I can recall few of their ministrations. There were relaxation exercises, of course. And at least one of them was interested in testing my cerebral dominance, my apparent right-handedness. I quickly spotted what she was up to and obliged her by saving myself with my left leg every time she tripped me up during solemn little walks round her office. It may even be that she wrote up my case history and it contributed to the 1950s popularity of mixed dominance as a factor in stammering.

Obviously, and regrettably, I didn't take the therapists I

was sent to seriously. I'm sure this wasn't because I didn't want to be cured. Of course I did – in the most ordinary conversations I was liable to twitch and jerk my head and stick my tongue out, and look so awful I was only too grateful when people averted their gaze. I hated stammering. No, the reason for my poor attitude towards the people who tried to help me was that the treatments they offered seemed so irrelevant . . . frankly, so *silly*. I knew very well how they could help me: they could teach me to recreate at will the sensation that came over me when I stepped on stage or opened the huge ceremonial bible in chapel. They never did. They never even tried. They tripped my feet and taught me bloody stupid relaxation exercises.

The sensation was very exact. I remember it, and the surrounding circumstances, with extraordinary vividness. I could isolate it particularly well in chapel, where I wasn't being chattered at by the stage manager or the director or other actors. As I sat awaiting the moment for the lesson I was going to read, my pulse increased not so much its rate as its intensity, its magnitude. It pounded in my ears and seemed to swell each vein and artery in my body. I would look at my hands, expecting to *see* them throbbing.

The prayer would end, or the hymn, or whatever – the exact rite escapes me, I haven't attended a church service in thirty years – and I would stand up in my seat, always conveniently at the end of a row, and walk up the aisle to the vast brass lectern. My feet would clack on the black-and-white tiles and I would be near to fainting with terror – no, not with terror, with excitement.

Beside the lectern there was a turn to the left and two steps up. I'd prepared the bible in advance, open at the right page, a marker by the beginning verse. Two curves of brass eagle wings projected beyond the top outside edges of the book and I gripped each one firmly, to stop my hands shaking. The scuffling and coughing of four or five hundred boys in the chapel settled down. I looked out across them, possessed by a terrible and perilous calm:

'Here beginneth the first lesson. The second book of Samuel, chapter one, verse twenty . . .'

My voice rang out, not a twitch, not a jerk, not a gasp or gargle, echoing back at me, reverberating among the pillars and dusty pinnacles of the organ case. But before I'd started, before I *could have* started, an essential change had taken place in the nature of my being. As I looked out across all the scrubbed faces and scruffy hair I felt it happen. I became no longer a stammerer.

The nearest equivalent I can find to the sensation is the delightful wave of drowsiness that a good sleeping pill induces in the one or two minutes before you actually nod off. It was like a beneficence. Not that I ever thought of it as God-given, even in those Christian days of my youth, but it descended over the cells of my brain, wafted blessedly through them, spread like a breath, lapped like gentling water.

If there were circuits wrongly connected, it reconnected them. If there were voltages set too high, it reduced them. If there were insecurities, fears, deprivations, it removed them. I was no longer a stammerer.

It descended like music. If there was a serpent in the house of my speech, the serpent slept, lulled by the music. And for as long as the water, the breath, the music wrapped me around, I wasn't a stammerer.

This doesn't mean I wasn't nervous. It doesn't mean I didn't fluff, make mistakes, lose my place like any other nice ordinary person. It simply means that for the duration of the second book of Samuel, or of the scene I was playing on the stage, the element of myself that made me a stammerer had gone away, been suppressed, somehow got cancelled.

Right afterwards, returned to my pew or backstage, in the wings and my whole self again, I'd stammer up a storm. But for the duration of the performance, whether on stage or at the lectern, not being a stammerer, I was someone else.

The ability to shed the crippling stammering persona, to step free of the stammer snake, isn't unusual. Actors, parsons in pulpits, even departmental managers in front of their departments, all sorts of stammerers have it. Personally, it only comes when the words I'm speaking aren't my own, but I gather that's my particular quirk. The important point, the point that's important for this present argument, is that stammers *can* be shed, even by severe sufferers, and nobody has the faintest idea how or why, and I think somebody ought to be trying to find out.

Various approaches suggest themselves. Are very young stammerers similarly affected by situation, by their emotional response to the speaker/audience relationship? If not, when does it begin to occur? Why? Also, since the adult ability to shed isn't universal, a comparative study of those who can and those who can't might be another good place to start.

Then again, if all the arty subjective stuff is stripped away from my above description of the shedding event, what's left sounds awfully electrical: maybe a sort of Dolby effect on the net of sparking synapses. A lot of research just now, in Massachusetts, is going into electroencephalographic studies of brain wave patterns at the moment of stammering – my suggestion is that a shift away to the beginning of the moment of not-stammering might also be useful. Then again, on the subject of this fluent speech in performance that many stammerers achieve – it fools audiences (who would have guessed, for example, that the marvellous stage delivery of Frankie Howerd was that of a stammerer?), but would it fool a properly set up analytical acoustic computer program? And if it didn't, might not constructive lessons be learned from the differences?

Maybe it's just that the lectern or the footlights conjure up a new, non-stammering identity. That's certainly part of what it feels like. As I look round an audience my knees bang together with stage-fright, my hands are clammy with the sweat of sheer terror and my bowels clamour for release . . . nevertheless, despite all this, there is absolutely no possibility that I will stammer. Forget my lines, yes. Exit left through a bookcase because I've forgotten where the door is, yes. Faint dead away, yes. But stammer – never. Stammering is what stammerers do and I'm not a stammerer. I've got a new identity.

So how is this new identity summoned up, what is it created out of, and why can't something other than footlights or lecterns do the job? Nobody knows. And my impression is, just at the moment, that nobody's trying to find out. Perhaps research into why people *don't* stammer seems a bit frivolous when we're still such a long way from knowing why they *do*, but I don't think it is. And it might turn out to be easier. There's no harm (only hundreds of thousands in non-existent research funds) in trying.

So that's my suggested new direction for future research. At the moment when a stammerer becomes a non-stammerer, a clear and predictable change occurs in him. It feels as if it occurs in his head, but maybe it really occurs in his elbow. In any case, with the timing of the event so exactly known, it shouldn't be impossible to run it to ground. To measure it. To hold it up to the light . . . To reproduce it clinically?

We live in a culture that has come to expect science to deliver cures for everything and to be outraged when it doesn't. Gradually we're learning the dangers of this attitude. Everything *isn't* curable, and I suspect that it's right that it shouldn't be, and perhaps stammering will turn out to be one of those disorders that remind us salutarily of our limitations. I hope not, though. That's a job for other people's disorders. Not mine or yours.

In the future, many wonders reside. UHF identity modulators, for a start. They'll do the job a treat, and who cares a damn about the ethics? For the moment, though, I hope the main thrust of this book has been positive, and optimistic. Even at the present imperfect state of our knowledge, stammering *is* remediable. Got at early enough, in the vast majority of cases this book has shown that it need never become established. And if it does, or if you're old like me, and a victim of Matthew Arnold and left foot tripping, there's still a lot that can be done. Therapies exist, good ones. And there are people to talk to, associations to join, many ways of taking away the isolation, the terrible sense of freakishness.

My speech is usually pretty good now. It improved steadily in my forties, due I'm sure to the blessings of a very happy marriage. Even so, there are still occasions in my life when nice (nasty?) ordinary people might be tempted to echo my mother's words and tell me, 'If I stammered as badly as you I wouldn't talk so much.' I'd see their point, too, because I do gab on sometimes, but I wouldn't take much notice. The stuff they have to put up with when faced with me is nothing to the stuff I have to put up with every day of my life, when faced with myself.

But in any case society's got much nicer these days (I do believe it has, you know, despite rising crime rates and bridge on TV), and I very seldom get any hassle. People are much more patient and reasonable than they were. Back in 1949, for example, in my National Service days, many of the corporals and sergeants seemed genuinely to believe that I was half-witted: they sniggered behind their hands, and explained things to me very slowly and loudly, using simple words and spacing them out to help me understand. I honestly don't think that, or anything like it, would happen today.

Not that the stammerer's lot will ever be easy. The Chronic Perseverative Speech Disfluency Syndrome hits him precisely where it hurts most: in what above all else makes him human, his speech. It may also jerk him about, outraging his autonomy. It's a heavy cross to bear. But at least he knows now that there are people on his side. There's an association looking after his interests, there's a medical profession sympathetic to his needs, and there are therapists able to help him. Also, and perhaps best of all, he knows that with the progress being made in the treatment of stammering in children there'll be steadily fewer people with his problems in the future.

A final note on my use here, for simplicity's sake, of the masculine pronoun. I shouldn't need to say that every word in this book applies just as much to girls and women as to boys and men. The female stammerer's burdens are just as great as the male's – perhaps in some respects greater, seeing that women start anyway from a position of enforced inferiority and low self-esteem in most of the world's societies. Her therapy, when on the world scale she's lucky enough to get it, is just as demanding. And her courage is just as impressive. So I can only hope that a matter of mere semantics hasn't made women stammerers feel excluded from this book. The same pious hope applies to the many male therapists who, by a similar simplification, I've written out of existence. The fault, really, lies with the English language, which is traditionally reluctant to see people as separate from their gender. But that's presumably because *people* are traditionally reluctant to see people as separate from their gender. And the reasons for that belong, alas, in another book.

Appendix 1

In the library of the Association For Stammerers is a unique and fascinating item of late Victorian stammering memorabilia, a turn-of-the-century book about the stammering schools of Mr Benjamin Beasley, and the Beasley System taught in them. Blatant promotion material, this book was privately produced by one W. J. Ketley, a Beasley son-in-law who had clearly taken over the London end of the operation and was running it with the help of his wife and their two daughters, Winnie and Gladys. It's fulsome stuff, of course, but I've edited it down to a reasonable length and I'm including it here for the sake of the revealing light it sheds on period attitudes, both to stammering and to children's upbringing in general.

On the subject of the System itself Mr Ketley is predictably discreet. 'Vocal Exercises' are vaguely referred to, and safe exhortations are made to 'keep cool and cultivate repose', but no trade secrets are revealed (the System is 'natural', by the way), and the bulk of the book is taken up with dire warnings to parents on the perils of delay in seeking treatment for their children's stammers, and glowing descriptions of the school buildings and their pastoral surroundings.

Today's Londoners will find it hard to recognise Willesden from these pages – water-fowl feature, and lowing cattle – but at least the author, torn between his potential customers' Rousseau-esque love of things rural and their liking for metropolitan convenience, does admit that his establishment is no more than four miles from Charing Cross, and within a five minute walk of Brondesbury station.

One or two stammering points are significant, however. Mr Ketley offers very un-Victorian (and good) advice to parents, combined with very Victorian (and bad) advice to stammerers – often via long hearty quotes from Charles Kingsley. The author has no opinion at all of rival 'systems' of course – in particular, if for decidedly odd reasons, of hypnotism. Clearly the hypnotists, following in Herr Mesmer's footsteps, were his most serious commercial threat.

Victorian snobberies are clear also. Most Beasley pupils are reassuringly described as being 'of the upper classes', while 'artizans' attend only in the evenings – at which time, however, their admirable ambition to better themselves provides incentive for an invariable cure.

On the other hand, when it comes to discussing fees, Mr Ketley is unashamedly populist: 'the scale of fees . . . is such as to bring the system of treatment within the reach of all classes of society'. Exactly how 'all classes of society' were expected to get on when meeting in his school's formidable Drawing Room (pictured below) is not gone into. I wonder, too, how 'all classes of society' will have responded to Mr Ketley's brisk advice concerning the choice of nurse or governess for the stammering child. Presumably, knowing the spirit of the time, with a becoming humility.

So now to Mr Ketley, of whom he tells us Mr Benjamin Beasley said, in an 1890 interview with one Raymond Blathwayte:

> My son-in-law, Mr W. J. Ketley, who superintends my house in London, and has studied and taught my system for twenty years, is even more patient than I am, and I feel that whenever I am obliged to give the work up it will be carried on just as effectually, if not indeed more so, as ever it has been in my own time . . .

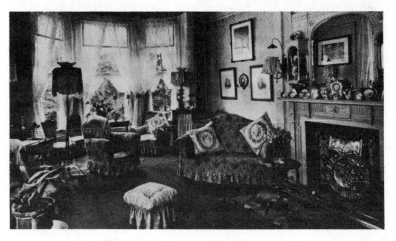

Tarrangower: Drawing Room

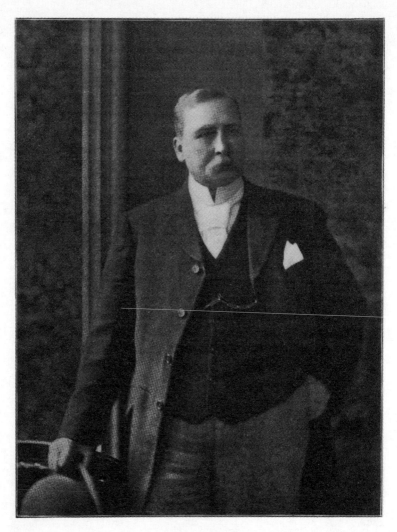

Mr. B. Beasley

THE BEASLEY SYSTEM

Perfected 1876.

ESTABLISHMENT FOR THE CURE OF STAMMERING AND ALL DEFECTS OF SPEECH

"TARRANGOWER,"

WILLESDEN LANE, BRONDESBURY, N.W.

For the reception of Resident and Non - Resident Pupils.

Principal: Mr. W. J. KETLEY, assisted by Mrs. Ketley (*née* Beasley) and the Misses WINNIE and GLADYS KETLEY.

"Tarrangower" is situated about 4 miles North West of Charing Cross and within five minutes' walk of Brondesbury Station.

Preface

In presenting this book to those whom it may concern, I desire to point out that since the deaths of the late Mr Benjamin Beasley and his son, the conduct of the Beasley system of treatment for the cure of stammering has fallen upon myself.

Before the late Mr Beasley made the discovery which eventually led to his cure, I was associated with him in business, and sympathetically watched the gradual process of his cure, aiding him with suggestions and talking over with him his difficulties until his impediment was entirely removed. I thus assisted him from the very first in the development of the system.

Having fully realised the value of that system, we disposed of our commercial enterprise and jointly took up the work of ministering to others. I was his constant companion, living in the same house, assisting in instructing the very first classes of pupils, aiding in the writing of his books, and helping in the elaboration of the exercises that were found necessary to meet the different forms of stammering and the different temperaments of stammerers who came to us for relief.

Later, when the growth of the business made extensions necessary, Brampton Park was taken for country pupils, and an establishment in London was opened, of which I have had sole charge for the past thirty years, and where I have given instruction to many hundreds of stammerers with complete success.

Tarrangower has been specially equipped for the reception of pupils of all ages. It is in a delightful district, within easy reach of the West End, and contains facilities for outdoor recreation, including tennis, and indoor amusements.

In conclusion, I wish to draw the attention of parents especially to the chapter on the Danger of Delay. The picture is by no means overdrawn; the stories that have been poured into my ears and the obvious effects of their impediment on many of the pupils who have ultimately come to me for relief having been heartrending. While the child is young the cure is easy; with those of mature years it is none the less certain, though greater watchfulness and care and more determination are necessary to obtain relief. And by that time great suffering has been endured.

In all cases the responsibility of parents is greater than they know, and for every one of those to whom this book may bring a fuller sense of that responsibility it will be some consolation to the writer to feel that at least an effort will be made to rescue a sensitive soul from a purgatory of living torment.

W. J. Ketley
Tarrangower,
178 Willesden Lane,
Brondesbury, N.W.

CHAPTER 1

Stammering: Its Handicap and Cause

To those afflicted with stammering there is only one subject of importance – their permanent cure. Their infirmity is an ever-present torment, marring the happiness of the present, blurring the visions and
destroying the ideals of the future. Few except those who do stammer
realise what an awful handicap in life the affliction imposes.

To the inveterate stammerer almost as many avenues of life are
closed as to the deaf and dumb. The army, the navy, the civil service,
public appointments, and public office of every kind, parliament, the
bar and the scholastic professions are sealed against them; while in
all the learned professions – the professions associated with the arts
and sciences – the inability to give vocal expression to their thoughts
and designs and discoveries is a drawback and an impediment to
progress.

In business it is the same. Bankers, merchants, stockbrokers, ship-
pers and manufacturers prefer to have in their business departments
men of facile speech. Even the stammering shopkeeper is unable to
explain the merits of his goods as he would wish, and as he knows
he could, but for the fatal lack of harmony between the nervous
system and the mechanical organs of speech, which locks his tongue.

In the humbler walks of life, too, the stammerer is debarred from
many callings. He can neither be railway guard, nor porter, nor
engine driver, nor policeman, nor soldier, nor jack tar. Only in the
most humble callings where silence is golden and physical work alone
is required, can he be said to feel least the restraint of his affliction.

Should he be tempted to go abroad, he may find the gates of
foreign countries closed against him as an emigrant, the example
having already been set by the United States, where inveterate stammering is held to be sufficient cause for refusing to its victim admission at the ports.

Yet among all men in the world there are none as a class who are
better equipped in mental ability, in versatility, in depth of pen-
etration, in nervous force, than the stammerer.

Carlyle, one of the keenest observers of his day, said that he never
knew a stammerer who was a fool. It is the nervous force, the intense
self-consciousness, the keen mental vitality of the patient, that in nine

cases out of ten leads to the partial breakdown of the harmonious association between the nervous and muscular mechanisms of speech, and gives rise to the impediment.

It must always be remembered that articulate speech is one of the most complicated of human achievements, requiring a series of nervous and muscular actions all of which must be executed with precision and in accordance. This is the baffling mystery of the affliction. It is not a disease. It is impossible for the physician to put his finger on any nerve or any part of the nervous system, or for the surgeon to point to any physical defect, and for either to suggest that by the stimulation of this nerve or the removal or amendment of that organ of speech a cure may be effected.

Neither drugs nor surgical treatment are of avail, and medical men are therefore prone to tell parents that the child will grow out of his infirmity. How hopelessly wrong they are ten thousand stammerers could bitterly explain.

But in the following pages it is demonstrated that no stammerer need remain the prisoner of his affliction. The history is given of an inveterate stammerer who, having borne his burden for over thirty years, effected his own cure and in so doing evolved a system which has been of incalculable benefit to thousands of stammerers and is still at the services of those who are harassed by one of the most distressing afflictions known to man.

CHAPTER 2

The Danger of Delay

One of the poets has told us that the pain and suffering wrought by want of thought exceeds in infinite volume that inflicted by want of heart. And, so far as the stammering child is concerned, no truer sentiment was ever penned.

If the mother and father of a stammering child only realised for one moment the possible life-long hell to which they were allowing their child to descend by neglecting the first symptoms of stammering, or refraining from taking advantage of the best opportunity offered for its cure, they would never forgive themselves. But their distress on first noticing the hesitation or the distinct stammer is in most cases lulled by the suggestion of a friend or the family doctor that the child will grow out of it. Would to Heaven there were any probability of this. But in not one case out of a hundred is the assurance made good by subsequent fact.

On the other hand, the hesitancy increases, the stammering becomes more pronounced, and though at home the child may seem cheerful and undisturbed, unconscious of its disability, no one except a stammerer knows how little truth there is in this seeming peace and indifference.

Only the stammerer knows the suffering endured even as a child, although protected and patiently borne with by loving parents; much less can anyone but a stammerer know the agony of being taken among strangers, or how soon the child learns to shrink from other children, how often he busies himself in looking out of windows or examining books when his heart is really at play with youngsters whom he would fain join but dare not.

Day by day, hour by hour, the consciousness of inability to speak as other children speak is there, the iron begins to enter into its soul, and the brighter and more intelligent and more sensitive the child may be, the deeper does its affliction wound.

When at length school days come to be talked of, the poor child, though it may put on a bold front, writhes in agony of mind. And when at last those school days materialise he learns to curse his halting tongue and to hate the dawn of every day because of the purgatory to which his fellows thoughtlessly condemn him. This is no fanciful picture. It is the true story of nine out of ten stammering children, whose sufferings sear their little souls each day.

Indeed, could fathers and mothers fully realise what the life of a stammerer means, no child would ever grow up to be a stammering man or woman. For once the child has become nervous, self-conscious, constrained, the hope that it will grow out of its affliction is vain, while the danger of delay remains, namely, that as it grows older the habit will become so ingrained that cure will be ten times more difficult.

The boy or girl taken in hand just before school age may be easily cured and sent to school free from the tyrant and rejoicing in the freedom of speech. The young man or young woman entering on the duties of life will find it more difficult to shake off the nervous dread of speech and change the conduct of their lives. Yet each is quite capable of cure, though greater perseverance may be demanded. But they need have no fear if they are steadfast, nor need either the man or woman of middle age, even though they have been stammering for the better part of a lifetime. It is never too late to mend, as Mr Beasley proved in his own case, and has been demonstrating in hundreds of cases since he opened his first establishment nearly forty years ago. There is the certainty of cure for any of them if they have sufficient determination to persist.

But undoubtedly the best time to tackle the affliction is in early youth, before the miseries of halting speech have wrecked the nerves. Until the child has reached an age at which he may be allowed to go from home, parents themselves can do much to help. The wisest course for them to pursue, as Mr Beasley himself taught, is to apparently take no notice of the impediment, but listen quietly and patiently, and themselves set an example by speaking slowly and thoughtfully. Care should be taken that any nurse or governess is of a calm and placid disposition, not likely to excite or hurry the child.

In its very early stages, therefore, every effort should be made to check the persistence of faulty speech, and should such treatment fail to secure the consummation so devoutly to be desired, then, when the time comes at which the child may be put under tuition, no time should be lost in obtaining the best aid possible.

The parent in making selection should be on his guard, taking care to satisfy himself that the system has no tricks, no extraneous aids, no suggestion of hypnotism or psychical influences, no medicines or physical operations, but is one that by natural means shall help the child to acquire self-control, concentration of thought, confidence in himself. These requirements the Beasley system fulfils in every detail, and it is because it does this that it has, during the past forty years, been so pre-eminently successful and so widely recognised, not only in the United Kingdom, but throughout the civilised world.

CHAPTER 3

Active Causes of Stammering

In our opening chapter it is pointed out that scientists have been quite unable to trace the impediment to any defect in the organs of speech. My own experience fully confirms this: during my intercourse with hundreds of stammerers I have never met with one whose impediment was so caused.

In addition to the mystery of the great underlying cause, however, there are four quite obvious principal active causes. First, not opening the glottis so as to produce sound; second, not allowing the lower jaw to have free play; third, pressing the lips tightly together; and fourth (a habit most difficult to get rid of), pressing the tongue tightly against the teeth or gums. In other words, stammering is caused by trying to speak in an impossible manner.

There are many secondary causes which first conduce to stammering, the diseases incidental to childhood being the principal, such as measles, scarlatina, whooping-cough, low fever, or anything which reduces the physical condition. Sometimes it is acquired by imitation. As a general rule it commences when children are between the ages of four and twelve years, and usually makes its appearance after recovery from some child-ailment. At first it is only slight, but does not take long to develop itself, and is often aggravated by the injudicious treatment of those having charge of children.

The absurd notion, which once had a few disciples, that stammering is a disease, has nearly become obsolete. To characterise as a disease an improper use of the lips, tongue, breath, and lower jaw seems quite as ridiculous as if speaking ungrammatically or biting one's nails were so called. Stammering is an affliction in which neither disease nor physical deformity has any part or share.

CHAPTER 4

Forms of Stammering

The phenomena of stammering are uncountably numerous and variable in form. The bad habits into which the lack of co-ordination in the mechanism of speech has driven the stammerer differ in every individual case; therefore individual treatment is essential.

Many cases have come under my own observation that could be quoted in proof of this. One gentleman, who finally came to me as a pupil and went away cured of his impediment, was often several minutes, making great efforts all the time, before he could utter a sound. When at last the sound came, ten or twelve words would be uttered with inarticulate rapidity until his breath was spent, whereupon he would be as long in trying to begin again. On one occasion, being asked a question by a friend with whom he was walking, he walked several hundred yards before replying, and when he did so the delay had been so long that his friend had forgotten what he had asked.

Another remarkable case, laughter-provoking were it not so piteous, was that of a young lady who, in her endeavours to speak, gave herself violent kicks, and had carried this so far, on her own telling, that on one or two occasions when out walking she had kicked or tripped herself into the gutter.

These are extreme cases, but nearly all stammerers distort their faces when attempting to speak, and hundreds get hold of bad mechanical habits. Some who are able to speak fairly to equals and superiors utterly fail to make themselves intelligible when speaking to servants. Most can at least speak passably in the family circle, but not at all in public. But at the present moment there is in the House of Lords an elderly nobleman who frequently inaugurates debates with perfect fluency, while in private conversation he stammers badly; and in a northern town the recent holder of the office of Mayor was a gentleman who, as a major in the volunteer force and as a public speaker was perfectly free of speech, while in private conversation he hesitated, stammered, and relapsed into silence because of his infirmity.

Opposite circumstances in other ways also have distinct effects. Some stammerers can speak with comparative fluency when conversing with strangers, but amongst their own friends experience considerable difficulty; while others find their troubles begin immediately they talk to anyone with whom they are unacquainted.

It is no easy matter for a stammerer to speak through a telephone or through a tube, as the knowledge that someone is listening at the other end is quite sufficient to upset him; while there are other stammerers who can use the telephone quite freely and yet be almost dumb when they meet face to face the person to whom they have spoken. It is often very trying for a stammerer to have to give his own name, or to be called upon to repeat anything he may have said, even though he had spoken it just before with perfect freedom.

It would take volumes to enumerate all such differences, and therefore only these must suffice.

CHAPTER 5

Stammering v. Natural Methods of Speech

Whatever may be the underlying cause of stammering, the active cause is evidently an attempt to speak in an impossible manner.

The ordinary man speaks without effort at all. His lower jaw is loose, his tongue and cheeks and lips are free and flexible, and his words flow easily and without exertion.

What the Beasley system teaches is the right, the natural method of speech. To this end three things are essential. That the stammerer be in good health, that he realises the necessity for both mental and physical repose, and that he has faith in himself. There is an old proverb which tells us that if money be lost naught is lost, if honour be lost much is lost, but that if courage be lost all is lost. It is undoubtedly so with the stammerer. If he loses courage, his case is hopeless.

But no stammerer with a spark of grit in his composition would permit himself to get into such a condition, and if he did, the sight of a class of stammerers – young, middle-aged and elderly – would surely help him to regain it, and would show him that if he is willing to try, and is ready to keep a watch on himself, and to endeavour to speak 'on rule' – that is, according to the methods of the Beasley system – his perfect cure is a matter of certainty.

First, then, the stammerer is taught to school himself to mental calm, to make no effort to speak until he feels in perfect mental and physical repose. Secondly, it is pointed out to him how utterly foreign to free speech is all effort, and how impossible it is for him to speak with clenched teeth, rigid jaw, or strained cheek and lips. The mechanism of speech permits of no such hard running; it should work smoothly and softly, and run like a well-oiled machine.

The Beasley system is designed to help stammerers to adopt only natural methods – to unlearn the bad habit of years, to discriminate between the impossible method and the possible, and so learn to speak naturally as men should.

The pity is that stammerers cannot be taught by printed instructions or correspondence. Each has his own peculiarities, and therefore requires to be dealt with individually. But more than that, he needs oral demonstration. In one oral and vocal lesson more can be taught than by days of reading and nights of study.

Indeed, the habit of speaking wrongly has become so much a part of the stammerer's nature that he is liable to wrongly interpret any printed or written instruction, and he will, in nine cases out of ten, find himself worse than when he attempted to speak before ever the lesson was scanned.

Moreover, without the stimulus of seeing the progress made by others who have been every whit as bad as he, the stammerer would find himself lacking the courage and self-control necessary to success. The meeting in class helps also to break through the reserve with which the stammering child so often surrounds himself, and encourages the sang-froid that is an essential part of the cure.

In brief, the system is a kindly, patient, watchful system of teaching the stammerer the true art of speaking; and because it is a natural system, built up by one who himself stammered, it contains such elements of success as cannot fail the pupil who is in earnest concerning his future welfare.

The great advantage of the Beasley system, and the one which gives it a pre-eminent claim to attention over all others, is that it was evolved by a gentleman who himself stammered for five and thirty years, who tried other systems without result and who, feeling with increased intensity as the years passed the seriousness of the handicap under which he laboured, determined to put all else aside and wrestle with his infirmity to a finish. His determination had its reward.

Inventing new vocal exercises and new expedients, unwearyingly analysing his every emotion, he continued casting about for a cure until a chance intonation in a vocal exercise gave him a hint, the full force of which, when he came to study the matter, flashed upon him like an inspired revelation. On that hint and inspiration he laboriously constructed his system and cured himself, to the wonderment of business acquaintances and the surprise and delight of his friends.

Of no other system can the same be said. Others may have been evolved as the result of much sympathetic study of stammerers, but it is safe to say that no one except a stammerer who has been taught by personal experience can enter into the emotions, the difficulties, and the terrors that the stammerer has to suffer and combat, or realise fully the essential cause of the affliction.

Since Mr Beasley had himself sustained heavy business losses because of his inability to present his views plainly to those with whom he was dealing, these aspects of the affliction were fully realised. In the workshop he had withdrawn from management because of the difficulty of giving clear instructions to the men; in the office he had withdrawn from all speaking parts, though knowing that in hundreds of business transactions he could have done infinitely better than those on whom the duty fell; and when at last he let all else go in order that he might study and cure himself, he found that these withdrawals of his had been among the errors that added to his infirmity, and realised that the building up of the nervous system, and the putting aside of the dread of association with other people, were two essentials necessary to success in overcoming the difficulties of his impediment.

In this his teaching is diametrically opposed to those whose instruction consists in insisting upon lengthened periods of silence, to be broken only in class or to the instructor, or in that much more insidious teaching which relies on hypnotic suggestion for the cure. In the one case the mechanism of speech is left idle instead of being usefully employed; in the other the will-power is being sapped, the nervous system weakened day by day, until the patient becomes but the puppet of the operator.

It is not the sapping of individuality that is necessary in the cure of the stammerer, but the contrary. Who that has dabbled with hypnotism at all has failed to note the class of persons that most easily come under the power of the hypnotist? Weak, inanimate, feeble creatures in physique, or if not this, then mentally dull, they represent the precise opposite of the ideal man or woman, and it were a sin against Heaven to sap the mental or physical health of even the most inveterate stammerer to effect what can at best be but a temporary cure of his one affliction.

The Beasley system is founded upon the opposite view. A sound mind in a sound body are its first essentials. And one of the first lessons his system teaches is that no one can cure a stammerer but himself. Once the subject realises this, and decides to profit by the instruction given, his cure is assured.

In no set phrase or polished paragraph can the Beasley system be better described than in the noble words of Charles Kingsley – himself a victim of the affliction:

'Let him (the stammerer) learn again the art of speaking, and having learned, think before he speaks, and say his say calmly, with self-respect, as a man who does not talk at random and has a right to a courteous answer. Let him fix in his mind that there is nothing on earth to be ashamed of save doing wrong, and no being to be feared save Almighty God, and go on making the best of the body and soul which heaven has given him, and I will warrant that in a few months his old misery of stammering will lie behind him as an ugly and all but impossible dream when one awakes in the morning.'

This is the Beasley system; it teaches the art of speaking, it induces self-respect, calmness, self-confidence, and where the patient himself is in earnest, it secures to him that freedom of speech which is to the stammerer above and beyond the gifts or the praises of Kings.

CHAPTER 6

A Product of Civilisation

Since speech in its higher forms is one of the most obvious finished products of civilisation, it is not surprising to learn that until they too were brought under the influence of civilised communities, stammering was unknown among the aborigines of Central Africa, the Redmen of North America, and the degenerate blacks of Australia. None have been known to stammer unless and until they have been touched by civilisation.

A curious feature about this fact is, however, that the stammering among these aborigines where it is manifest at all does not arise from the greater complexities, the wider range, or the vaster number of words in the vocabulary of the civilised peoples with whom they have come in contact compared with the linguistic poverty of their native tongue, but rather from the causes that have played their part in the encouragement of the higher civilisation of which the scientific and poetic vocabulary is the hallmark. In other words, there is little or no language difficulty in the way of, or to account for, the stammerer.

It must be admitted, however, that in Spain and Italy stammerers are few, and this, it has been argued, may arise from the soft, easy flow of the Latin tongue. The suggestion, however, is hard of belief in view of the fact that in France, where the language of the people also owes much to the Latin tongue, stammering is quite as common as in Great Britain.

The key to the situation is, perhaps, to be found near home. In Ireland, we are told on the authority of the late Sir William Wilde, that stammering is much more common in the north than in the south. Now, the north of Ireland is noted for its industrial activity, while in the south the pastoral habits of the people have much in common with the every-day existence of the ease-loving Spaniard and Italian. *Mañana, Mañana* – tomorrow, tomorrow – is as much the ejaculation of the man of the south of Ireland as it is of the Spaniard. And tomorrow is often long in coming.

In the great mills and shipyards of Belfast, however, there are no yesterdays and no tomorrows. Life is just one perpetual Now, and the rush and wear and tear of industrial strife is responsible for the neurosis which predisposes so many more people to stammering – as also to other nervous ills – in these particular districts than in the less strenuous pastoral areas of the country, where the parents are connected with agricultural or other outdoor pursuits and are slower in speech, more deliberate in action, so that their children learn to speak slowly too.

Nor is this all. Civilisation carries with it many other factors predisposing to neurotic affections when regarded in comparison with the lives of savages who are brought up amid surroundings and conditions of perfect freedom.

Some philosophic soul has said that 'When the monkey blushed man was born.' Whether this be true or not, it undoubtedly is true that when man first blushed the stammerer came into being. Blushing, nervous dread, hesitation are all steps towards stammering, and all are due to the repressive influences of civilisation, with all its erotic and neurotic tendencies. The child of the savage is brought up like a healthy little animal, with all the facts of life exposed to him, recognising nothing in the crudities of life that would bring even the faintest blush to his cheek.

How different is the every-day training of the child brought up in a civilised environment — taught to whisper of the most intimate things, to disguise his real instincts, to ask for what he wants as a privilege instead of taking it as a right, to learn lessons instead of gambolling in the fields. And so, his animal spirits and vitality being kept in check, neurotic conditions are engendered. And finally, where the temperament is especially highly strung, and the predisposing conditions exist, he becomes a stammerer — a victim of civilisation.

We are told that industrialism wears out a family in three genera-tions, and those who know anything of our great industrial centres will be the last to dispute this statement. If the conditions under which we live thus destroy the physical frame, how much more likely are they to play havoc with the vastly finer and more sensitive ner-vous system? Stammering is thus undoubtedly one of the penalties that civilised people have to pay for their luxuries and refinements; and it rests on us to show that this same civilisation can come to the rescue of its own victims, and restore them to the full measure of the power of the inheritance to which they were born.

CHAPTER 7

An Independent Witness

A multitude of independent witnesses could be summoned to bear testimony to the thoroughness of the Beasley system, but perhaps the following report of a visit paid by Mr Raymond Blathwayte to headquarters will suffice:

> The evening shadows were lengthening over the broad swards and green lawns of Brampton Park as I drove up the long entrance to the beautiful old house, with its quaint gables and elaborately carved chimneys. A flight of water fowl winged their way to some distant mere, the lowing of cows was in the air, and a charming rural quietude greeted me, fresh from the roar and bustle of Piccadilly Circus.

My host, genial and sportsmanlike to his fingertips, came forward to meet me, and I caught a glimpse of some well-set-up young fellows with guns upon their shoulders disappearing in the direction of the stables. The whole place breathed that atmosphere of sport so delightful to the healthy, well-regulated English gentleman. I thought to myself, 'Nothing scholastic, nothing of the pedant here,' as I entered the great hall, in which two or three good-looking girls and a man or two were knocking about billiard balls.

'We don't go in very much for the ordinary scholastic life here,' said Mr Beasley, as we sat down in his study and lit our cigars. 'I like my young people of both sexes to feel that they are at home. They are mostly of the upper classes, and life here is very much what it would be in any well-regulated English home, with the addition of careful tuition. At the same time, the course of study here is very strict, and the hours are fully as long as they are at Eton or Harrow. Those young people whom you saw enjoying themselves in the hall just now have had a good hard day's work.

'I like to catch the stammerer young,' humorously continued Mr Beasley, 'although stammering is a thing that can be cured at any age. I am myself a remarkable instance of the possibility of stammering being cured late in life, for till I was forty years of age my existence was rendered quite unbearable by this unfortunate habit. But despite my own case, I like to catch the stammerer when he is young, and devote two or three years to curing his habit . . .

'But there's the dinner bell: and you must come and be introduced to my wife and my pupils. For it is mainly due to my dear wife that I have been so successful. No one, not even myself, has benefited my pupils in every respect so much as she has.'

A little while after dinner – which was very much like the festive meal at an ordinary big country house – we all assembled in the music room for the evening's entertainment.

The first item in the programme was a recitation charmingly delivered by a young fellow fresh from Eton. 'Now, there,' whispered my host, 'is a young fellow who six weeks ago could scarcely speak. He has gone in for my system heart and soul, with the result that he now speaks almost perfectly.'

'Yes,' I replied, 'but what a splendid elocutionist he is.'

'Ah, that is part of my system,' answered Mr Beasley. 'I make a point not only of curing the stammer, but also of perfecting speech.'

Then a young man got up and gave us a short, bright dissertation on dreams. He did it admirably and humorously, standing upon an elevated platform, Mr Beasley himself seated opposite him. 'Slowly, slowly,' cried the master of the house. 'Remember what I said this morning. Keep cool and cultivate repose. You will think and speak the better if you are perfectly at rest.'

A little boy of twelve then gave an address in a manner which rendered it difficult to believe that only a few months before he had been unable to answer a question of the most simple nature. Mr Beasley himself wound up the evening's performances with a recitation from Tennyson, his elocution charming, his delivery of the melodious lines smooth and gliding and unhesitating.

On the following morning Mr Beasley took me over the beautiful house and wide-spreading park. It is situated about a mile and a half from Huntingdon, and close to the River Ouse, where good fishing and boating are easily available.

When we entered the great class-room, where the pupils were all assembled, awaiting us, I was keenly interested in the exercise which followed. I cannot divulge the system – it would not be fair to Mr Beasley, although as a matter of fact it would be impossible for any outsider, not thoroughly acquainted with the inner meaning of the system, to attempt to teach it. I was also much interested in a book used in the class, in which the whole of the elementary formations of the English language are embodied in one chapter, so that every day the pupils are put through a thorough course, scientifically adapted to help them to overcome their affliction.

Nothing but personal contact with his many and varied types of stammerers has helped Mr Beasley to his success. He adapts his system individually, feeling that the method which might be successful with one person would utterly fail with another. But stammerers may rest assured that a few weeks' personal aid from him, backed up by firmness on their part, will inevitably result in their complete cure.

This, then, is the Beasley system. I cannot give better advice to those of my pupils who already know it than that they supplement it by the following words, taken from an article by Mr Charles Kingsley in *Fraser's Magazine*:

Stammerers need above all to keep up that which is nowadays called somewhat offensively 'muscular Christianity' – a term worthy of a puling and enervated generation of thinkers who prove their own unhealthiness by their contempt of that health which ought to be the normal condition of the whole human race.

But whosoever can afford an enervated body and an abject character, the stammerer cannot. With him it is a question of life and death. He must make a man of himself, or be liable to his tormentor to the last.

Let him, therefore, eschew all base perturbations of mind: all cowardice, servility, meanness, vanity, and hankering after admiration; for all these will make many a man, by a just judgment, stammer on the spot. Let him, for the same reason, eschew all anger, peevishness, haste, or even pardonable eagerness. Let him eschew, too, all superstition, and all which can weaken either nerves or digestion; all intemperance in drink or in food, remembering that it is as easy to be unwholesomely gluttonous over effeminate hot slops and cold ices as over manly beef and beer.

Let him avoid all else which will injure his wind and his digestion, and let him betake himself to all manly exercises. Let him, if he can, ride and ride hard; let him play rackets and fives, row and box. Above all, let him box, for so will the noble art of self-defence become to him a healing art.

If he doubt this assertion, let him hit out right and left for five minutes at a point on the wall as high as his own face (hitting not from the elbow like a woman, but from the loin like a man) and he will soon become aware of his weak point by a severe pain in the epigastric region in the same spot which pains him after a convulsion of stammering.

And let him now, in these very days, join a rifle club, and learn in it to carry himself with the erect and noble port which ought to be the common habit of every man. Thus, physically fit, the stammerer is able to tackle his infirmity under fair conditions. His body and mind vigorous and clear, he can fight the enemy that has so long oppressed him and, if he is really in earnest, will come out the victor.

Terms

Mr Ketley wishes it to be clearly understood that the scale of fees charged and the arrangements made for giving instruction are such as to bring the system of treatment within the reach of all classes of society.

No charge is made for consultation, and it is eminently desirable, in the best interests of the prospective pupil, that a personal interview should be arranged when information as to terms is being sought. Much depends on the temperament of the individual and the character of the impediment, and the consequent probabilities concerning the time necessary to effect a cure in each case.

Many artizans and tradesmen have been treated at evening classes with the most satisfactory results, and their ambition to rise in the world has proved a great incentive to effort which has resulted in complete success. For such pupils apartments near by are recommended as tending to a considerable reduction in expense.

Stammerers are treated either with or without scholastic instruction, but where the latter is required parents are assured that the
pupil will receive a thoroughly sound education.

Public School Boys received during their holidays.

Undergraduates can study and be coached during vacation while
being treated for their stammering.

Stammerers past middle life have been treated with unqualified
success, and many cases which have defied all previous attempts at
cure have succumbed to the Beasley system. These satisfactory results
can only be traced to the Extreme Simplicity of the system, which
in itself compels perfect action of speech, and makes the pupil a
Better Speaker than the majority of those who have never stammered.

Testimonials

For obvious reasons these are not printed in this volume, but many
hundreds of letters from old pupils may be seen at Tarrangower,
and lists of up-to-date references will be sent on application.

Appendix 2

Useful addresses and telephone numbers.

AFASIC (The Association for All Speech Impaired Children)
347 Central Markets
Smithfield
London EC1A 9NH
Tel: 071-326-3632

The Association For Stammerers
St Margaret's House
21 Old Ford Road
London E2 9PL
Tel: 081-983-1003

The College of Speech and Language Therapy
Bath Place
Rivington Street
London EC2A 3DR
Tel: 071-613-3855

The European League of Stuttering Associations
c/o BV Stotterer-Selbsthilfe
Kasparstrasse 4
D-5000 Köln 1
Germany

The International Fluency Association
Box 870242
Tuscaloosa
Alabama 35487-0242
USA

National Stuttering Project
4601 Irving Street
San Francisco
CA 94122-1020
USA

Speakeasy (The Association of Speech Impaired)
34 Newark Street
London E1 2AA
Tel: 071-377-7177

Speech Foundation of America
PO Box 11749
Memphis
Tennessee 38111-0749
USA

VOCAL (Voluntary Organisations Communication And Language)
336 Brixton Road
London SW9 7AA
Tel: 071-274-4029

Bibliography

BLOODSTEIN, O., *A Handbook on Stuttering*, Chicago: National Easter Seal Society, 1987.

BOOME, E. J. and RICHARDSON, M. A. (eds), *The Nature and Treatment of Stuttering*, London: Methuen, 1931.

BROWN, B. B., *Speech Therapy: Principles and Practice*, Edinburgh: Churchill Livingstone, 1981.

BYRNE, R., *Let's Talk About Stammering*, London: Association For Stammerers, revised edition, 1991.

CARLISLE, J. A., *Tangled Tongue*, Toronto: University of Toronto Press, 1985.

CURLEE, R. F. and PERKINS, W. H. (eds), *Treatment of Stuttering: New Directions*, San Diego: College Hill Press, 1984.

EMERICK, L. L. and HAMRE, C. E. (eds), *An Analysis of Stuttering*, Danville: Interstate, 1972.

FRANSELLA, F., *Personal Change and Reconstruction*, London, New York: Academic Press, 1972.

GLAUBER, I. P., *Stuttering: A Psychoanalytic Understanding*, New York: Human Sciences Press, 1982.

INGHAM, R. J., *Stuttering and Behavior Therapy*, San Diego: College Hill Press, 1984.

IRWIN, A., *Stammering: Practical Help for All Ages*, Harmondsworth: Penguin Books, 1980.

IRWIN, A., *Stammering in Young Children*, Wellingborough: Thorsons, 1988.

McCRONE, J., *The Ape That Spoke*, London: Macmillan, 1990.

MUIRDEN, R., *Stammering Correction Simplified*, London: J. Garnett Miller, 1971.

NEWARK, T., *Not Good At Talking*, Bath, London: Barton Books, 1985.

RIPER, C. Van, *The Treatment of Stuttering*, New York: Prentice-Hall, 1976.

ROCKEY, D., *Speech Disorder in 19th-Century Britain*, London: Croom Helm, 1980.

RUMSEY, H. St J., *The Stammerer's Choice*, London: Methuen, 1950.

St LOUIS K. O. (ed), *The Atypical Stutterer*, Orlando: Academic Press, 1986.

WALL, M. J. and MYERS, F. L., *Clinical Management of Childhood Stuttering*, Baltimore: University Park Press, 1984.

WILSON, J., *Self-Help Groups*, London: Longman, 1986.

———, *To the Stutterer*, Memphis: Speech Foundation of America, n.d.

Index